The Stroke

That Changed My Life

By Frank Hegyi

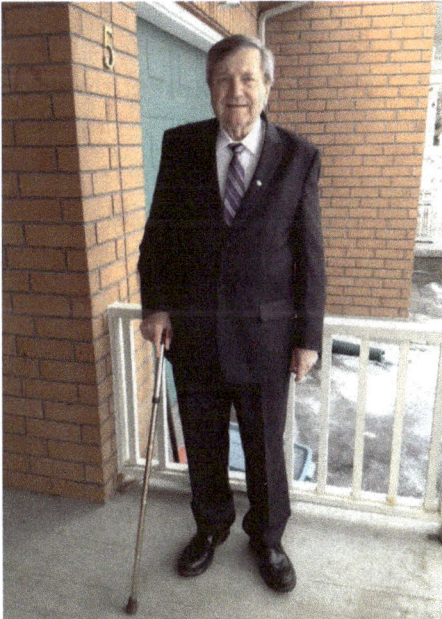

cistel

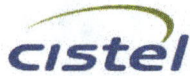

For partial financial support for the project
and
The Civic Campus, Saint Vincent Hospital,
Bruyere Hospital and Aphasia Centre
for expert medical care

Published by

Frank Hegyi Publications
1240 Kilborn Place, Unit 5
Ottawa, Ontario
Canada K1H 1B4

www.hegyipublications.com

© Frank Hegyi – 2012

ISBN 978-0-9812495-4-4

Dedication

I dedicate with book to my wife, Rose Hegyi, for her commitment to stay with me in my difficult time. After passing out in the hospital on the first day, I was not able to communicate until 4 weeks later. Once I did, my vocabulary was limited to 20 words. When I said "Hi" to Rose, she embraced me with a smile. My loving wife visited me in the hospital for 5 months, and she is constantly looking after me.

Acknowledgments

I had difficulty writing this book. I started in January 2012, and I had to make spelling corrections to each sentence. I have published 3 books before this one, but the language difficulty in this project was significant.

The following people have helped me with the language. My friends: Rose Hegyi (my wife) and Dr. Venkat Narasimhan, who edited the text, fixed the grammar and corrected the spelling mistakes. I am grateful to Jennifer (my daughter), Randy (my son) and his fiancée Sharon and Michael Hegyi (my son) and his wife Penny and daughter Tassia, who also helped with the language.

I am especially grateful for the staff of Civic Campus, Saint Vincent Hospital, Bruyere Hospital and Aphasia Centre for expert medical care.

Finally, I need to thank Dr. Nishith Goel and Cistel Technology for getting me back to work.

TABLE OF CONTENTS

INTRODUCTION

The bad day came into my life on February 19th 2011. I was having breakfast with my daughter and she observed me picking up the paper aggressively. My daughter, Jennifer, asked my wife to look at what I was doing; they realized that I had suffered a stroke. Jennifer helped me walk out to the car, and my wife and two grandchildren sat in the back seat as we headed to the hospital. I had a far-away look, and I did not realize what was happening to me.

Within an hour I lost consciousness, and I did not communicate for 4 weeks. When I regained my faculties, I was communicating with only a 20-word vocabulary, my right side was partially paralyzed, I could not sit up, and the doctors told my wife that I could be a vegetable.

While I could not speak, I did understand some of what was said to me; in particular, I zeroed in on the words the doctors told my wife to be a vegetable.

This story describes my fight.

STROKE

On February 19th 2011 I was at home waiting for my daughter to come over for breakfast. It was the day before my grandson's 8th birthday; after breakfast we were planning to shop around for his birthday present. During breakfast, my daughter, Jennifer, observed me looking at the paper aggressively. When she asked me what was the matter, I was not responding, just stared in a feeling of helplessness.

Jennifer jumped in to give me support, and I was gradually losing consciousness. My wife Rose helped Jennifer escort me into the car:

I was suffering from a stroke.

The hospital was about 20 minutes from my home. My two grandchildren piled in the back seat with my wife, and I was sitting in the front seat with Jennifer doing the driving. During the trip to the hospital, I was at peace with the world; it was very quiet. From the front seat I could see the world outside, and it gave me an uneasy feeling. As we got

9

into the hospital, my daughter grabbed a wheelchair and quickly wheeled me to the emergency room. Within minutes I was in a flatbed with the paramedics driving me to a special hospital for stroke patients, which was half an hour away. My wife came with me in the ambulance, while my daughter drove the children to a friend's house who could look after them. She then followed us to the hospital. So she could look after them while she was following us to the hospital.

It was quite a struggle for my daughter. Just a month before that her husband passed away due to cancer. She was counting on me to help her with the children, Ryan was 7 and Sara was 6 years old. Now, I was taken to the hospital, the same one where my son-in-law had had the operation before the cancer progressed to the brain. Due to the fact that I have a heart condition, I ended up in the same ward my son-in-law had been in just a few months earlier. I was familiar with cancer; in 2004 I was suffering from

Prostate cancer, had radiation treatment, and now this: a Stroke.

By the time Jennifer came to the hospital, I had lost consciousness. Yet, within an hour and a half, I had received an injection critical to life. I lay in the bed, tubes hanging in my mouth and nose, drifting in and out of consciousness. I felt a bit of pain, but only semi-consciously. Rose told Jennifer that I had lost consciousness, and the Doctors and nurses had their work cut out to fully bring me back. I did not recognise Rose or Jennifer. Jennifer then called my son, Mike, in Madison, who was ready to come the next day. Then, Rose called Randy from Orillia, and he was ready to come over. My wife stayed by my side all night, and the nursing staff really looked after me. By next morning, Mike had arrived. The following day my daughter in-law and my granddaughter arrived, and they were making conversation to me, but I was barely responsive. Then, my other son Randy arrived, and I did not recognize him either. My family, deeply worried, kept trying to communicate with me, but I barely understood what they were saying. I lay there, barely conscious, just drifting. I felt the presence of family around me, but I could break through from my world to them.

Within a week, a doctor told my wife that she should get used to my "vegetative" existence; if I even survive, it will be permanent. What I had suffered was a severe stroke, and I may even end up partially paralyzed. By the second week, my family was told that it was doubtful that I would even survive. My condition was worsening, and the Doctors induced "stroke" like existence, by putting me into a coma. I was in that state for a week, and after that they nursed me back to a semi-conscious state. In this state, I could not recognize anybody, but lay in a vegetative malaise. My daughter tells me that I utilized every piece of life support equipment the room had to offer.

A few days later, my wife and son (Randy) went to see my business partner Nishith Goel, and he was told about my condition. He told Rose that I would survive, and that he would support me any way he could. Nishith assured Rose that my office will be waiting for me to return to work, that the company was running smoothly. He was very supportive of my family, and called Rose every week for a status update. I understood that, and it was reassuring that he wanted to get me back to work. I was a scientist, author of over 35 publications, co-writer of a book and speaker in scientific conferences. I was a high profile member of the company; I had a contract with the Ministry of Natural Resources and with the Armed Forces, and I was doing the company research and development work. I had travelled to many different countries; in the past decade alone I had travelled 14 times to India. Previously, I travelled to Hungary (my native country) where I had an office and a manufacturing facility; to Russia on consulting

13

business; to China for project evaluation; Argentina for proposed business and Brazil for project management. We had an international company, and I did most of the consulting worldwide. In Canada I ran the research and development aspect of the company. I went from that to a stroke victim, who the doctors said would be a permanent vegetable.

About 14 days later, my wife called the priest so he could pray for me. I seemed to recognize the priest and would distantly respond to his prayers. In those moments, I could see Rose praying with the priest, which was very comforting to me. While I was not able to communicate with my family, I had a vague sense that I would hang in there. The presence of the priest was the first thing I recognised after the stroke. I sensed his compassion as he was there quietly praying with Rose. Even though I could not communicate with people, I received comfort from the support of my family.

After the priest's visit, I could hear people's voices, but their words were incomprehensible to me. I heard the doctor tell my wife that I would be vegetable, confined to bed, unable to feed myself, escort myself to the washroom, that I would need constant care. I was aware of the discussion around me but I could not respond in any way.

Recovery was very tough those first 4 weeks in the hospital. My family was there, all around me, but I could not reach out or respond to them. My grandchildren were there, but they could not understand my struggle to survive. My movements were limited, and, at times, it felt like my arms and legs were paralyzed. I kept trying to remove the annoying tubes from my mouth, but the nurses put them back in place so I could get some air. It was frustrating for me during this time because I was in the world, I saw everyone around me, my family, the medical staff, but I was unable to interact with them in any way. I was only semi-conscious, wishing to communicate, but my mouth would not cooperate. If I did attempt to speak, the words were garbled, and did not come out right.

But, after about 4 weeks, I opened my eyes and saw Rose holding my hand. Suddenly the word, "Hi", just leapt from my mouth, and Rose was very excited by this communication, hardly able to believe that I had actually said hello. She called the nurse over, and they talked to me. I vaguely understood what they were saying, and I tried to say a few more words. One of the first things I was able to express was to enquire how long I had been in the hospital. When Rose told me four weeks, I could hardly believe that much time had elapsed. My limited vocabulary was only about 20 words, but I could communicate. I could understand almost everything people were saying, but my vocabulary had taken quite a beating. When people spoke directly to me, I often understood what they were saying; but was not able to translate meaning from pictures I was shown. The day I was able to finally move my toes, I was extremely relieved and happy to find I was completely paralyzed. There was a bit of hope for me. Yet paralysis had affected my speech, and my mobility was greatly reduced.

I could hardly wait to see the Doctor. When I asked about my condition, he was not very optimistic, as he told me of the obstacles I would have to face. He said I had suffered a serious stroke, which had impacted the blood vessels on the left side of my brain, as well as my motor skills, which are governed by the right side of the brain. While there may be variations as to the extent of the damage, it appeared I would have limited right-side movement, as well as speech deficiency. When asked to lift my leg, I could only lift my toes, and only my right hand would move. The Doctor asked the nurses to move me to a wheelchair. This was achieved by wrapping me in a blanket attached to a lift, which gently raised me out of bed and moved me over to the chair. I found this incredible: how is it that I could not move, that I could only just lie there while all of this was done for me? After being lifted to the chair for the first time, I got very tired within a half-hour and had to be returned to bed. As time went by, I could extend the time out of bed to an hour before having to return. As I lay there in bed, I thought about my vegetative state: no movement in my leg, limited left side arm movement, having to be assisted by two people just to make it to the toilet. I did not want to be like that. At that time, I decided that I would do anything to get out of my bed and be able to walk again. I then asked Rose and Jennifer to push me around the ward, as I looked through the windows at the sunny world outside. It was spring. I had entered the hospital in winter, and now it was spring.

While in the hospital I saw other patients confined to wheel chairs and their beds. This was their entire world, and the doctors predicted that it would be mine, too. However, I was not ready or willing to merely accept the doctor's prediction; I was whole-heartedly fighting this.

But, at the moment, I had to face reality: I was lying in bed, partially paralysed. Many people in this condition suffer suicidal ideation, but in my case I did not, which I attribute to the strong support of my family. This is something I would always remember.

At the end of March, the hospital transferred me to Saint Vincent hospital, which accommodated invalid patients. And, I was, indeed, treated as an invalid. The hospital was packed with wheel chairs; the only ones mobile were the nurses, hospital staff, and visitors who came to see the patients.

At the new hospital, I had a double room all to myself. I had arrived there by ambulance, along with my wheel chair and bed lift. The trouble was, my feet were not cooperating at all, and I could only stay in the wheel chair for a maximum of 2 hours before needing to return to bed. Initially I required two attendants to lift me out of bed or take me to the toilet, and nursing staff had to feed me. I would just lie there in bed, hardly able to move my leg. However, the doctor told my wife that I was recovering well and that there was some hope that I would not remain in a vegetative state. This was welcome news to me, and gave me hope that I would one day walk again. My wife was visiting me every day except Sunday, and on those days my daughter and grandchildren came to visit. The first Saturday I was there, a Sister came to see me, and when she realized that I was Catholic, she invited me to Sunday Mass. When I expressed my interest in going, my wife offered to take me. That Sunday I woke up early, two people lifted me out of bed and into the wheel chair, where I ate my breakfast, and then I was ready to go to church. Within 15 minutes of the service, my wife was there by my side, and even the Sister showed up to assist as I was wheeled from my room. I was in a room on the 4th floor, and the church service was held two floors up, on the 6th floor. Of course, it was full of wheel chairs; my wife pushed me to the second row, but she sat to the side of the room; only the patients were allowed to sit in the rows down the middle of the room. The priest was assisted by the Sisters. It was a traditional mass, and at the time of the communion, the Priest came to each person to offer the blessing and the bread. All I could think of during the Mass was getting up and walking again. But so far, only my toes and one part of my leg were moving. Mass lasted one hour, and afterwards we left for our room. When we got there, I asked for help getting into bed, as I was exhausted from using up so much energy during the service.

When I was alone in bed, I visualized walking again. I tried to put my legs and arms into motion. It was hard but I started to have hopes that I would walk again. I practised for about half an hour each day, and I began to experience greater mobility. I was able to practice quite a bit with my arm, but the leg would require more time.

The next Monday the nurse came in with two people to see me; they were physiotherapists, one specialized in movement, the other in speech. This was the start of physical therapy. They scheduled me for some exercises. First I had a session with the speech therapist. The result was interesting. I looked at pictures and tried to describe their meaning, but was not able to for several of them. I recognized the pictures and the word for it when the therapist said it, but I was not able to articulate it myself. What this told me is that my vocabulary was greatly reduced by the stroke, but I had retained most of my comprehension skills.

In the exercise room, I had to face reality as well. It took a strong effort just to move my legs. I found I could move my left leg with some assistance, but my right arm and leg were almost totally unresponsive. The exercise therapist, Chantelle, was very helpful and encouraged me to keep trying. I looked forward to the sessions with her, and I felt I was improving. She was gentle but firm, as she looked after my needs. Chantelle was there to assist me into my wheel chair and help me exercise, during which time. I was able to see actual improvement as a result of my efforts.

This experience reminded me of an earlier episode I had had with paralysis. When I was 32 years old (two years after Rose and I got married, 38 years ago) I was diagnosed with Mary Strumpell spondylitis or Ankylosing spondylitis. Ankylosing spondylitis is a very painful and debilitating arthritis of the spine. Untreated it can lead to permanent fusing of the spinal column. Other ailments associated with Ankylosing spondylitis include Iritis, Plantar Fasciitis, Anemia, and loss of energy. When you see a bent over man or woman, they are suffering from spondylitis.

At the age of 32, I was potentially a life-long cripple, with a progressive illness that could leave me wheel-chair bound in as little as a year. I had some

23

thinking to do. The job I had at the time as a Forest Engineer required me to be outside much of the time, covering samples of jack pine trees and burning the leaves and branches for dry matter weight. In a wheel chair I would be unable to perform the necessary job requirements. I had taken a Master's Degree in Science, so I could have a job in the dry matter production, where I studied specific gravity of trees. Further, I studied the dry matter distribution of trees within the bole and between trees. After careful consideration, I decided to halt my field work, and take up statistics instead. This is something I could do even from a wheel chair. This was the first time in my life that I had ever faced a physical limitation, and I had to ask my wife to drive me to the office. I was a scholar of statistics and now my life has taken yet another turn; I had gone from field work, to the book study of a statistical scholar. My wife was beside me the entire time, driving me to the office every day, and picking me up after work. After a few months, I found my legs getting stronger, and I was able to begin walking with a cane. It took a lot of work to condition my legs, and even just standing took a lot of effort, but I was determined. I could stand up; I could move my legs, and I would gradually learn to walk again. The illness lasted about a year, and during that time I continued to improve at walking. Due to my speedy recover, a doctor referred me to a study questioning my initial diagnosis. The study conducted by a group of doctors determined that I had in fact had Mary Strumpell spondylitis, but had made a recovery through hard work and determination. I felt maybe that it was mind over matter, and this encouraged me to get out of my present paralysis.

I found the present challenge more than a little daunting, as I lie there partially crippled in a hospital bed after doctors have told my wife that I may be in a permanent vegetative state. This was a greater challenge than what I had previously face. I would I would walk again, but it was going to require a lot more effort and determination.

THE FAR AWAY WORLD

At an early age, I was influenced by my grandfather, who told me of the big wide world far away, where people live happily. It was my dream to go there, and when I got scolded I just wanted to run away to that wonderful place. At the age of three, my mother scolded me, and I had her pack me a bag of sandwiches so I could run off to the "big world."

The village priest who took this picture of me (Figure 1), asked me if there was a big world; with child-like confidence I replied that it was in the next village, where my god mother lives. As I was watching the camera, the priest told me that birds would fly out when the picture was taken. It was his way of entertaining a young boy who had to get his picture taken. The village priest was a photographer, who developed a lot of pictures of our village in happier times. The picture he took of me was shown in an exhibition in later years.

My mother, who had been watching from the window as the priest took my picture, came to escort me home, with the priest's soft laughter echoing behind us.

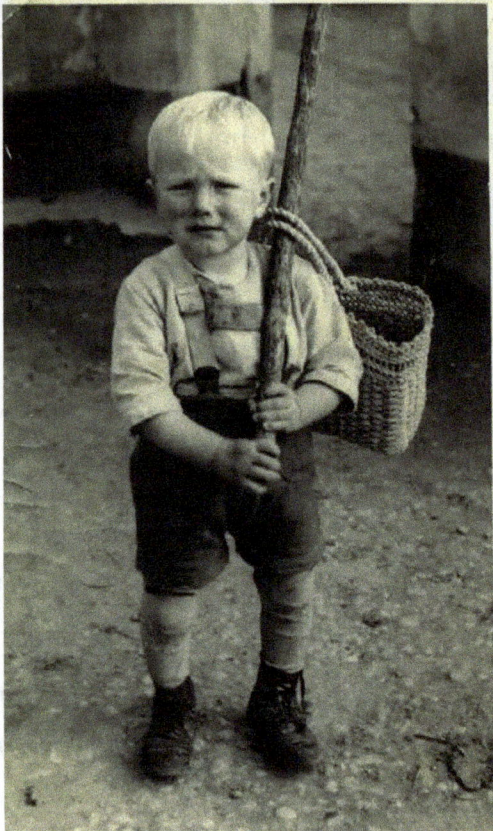

Figure 1: Frank is off to the "big world".

I grew to adulthood in the village, and my grandfather continued to be a major influence to me over the years. He took me to watch the cows grazing and told me stories about the big world. He made it all sound so real that I almost felt I was there, watching people going to work, play on the playground, go to bed, and wake up in the morning to do it all over again.

During the end of the Second World War, the military at the front came through our village and we had to hide in an underground bunker. My father and grandfather dug a bunker in the backyard and covered it; we used straw for blankets. I was 5½ years old and already had to learn the lesson of survival. If ever we heard anyone in the backyard, we had to stay still and quiet so the soldiers would not discover us.

My father went out whenever possible to care for the livestock and our possessions. One day a Russian soldier tried to steal our horse, and my father challenged him. They wrestled in the grave yard, and my father was spared from being shot only by the intervention of my grandfather, who handed the horse over to the soldier. My grandfather said the war was a cruelty the politicians subjected us to just to make us suffer more. The fact is, although I was only a young child, it did open my eyes to the reality and scope of human suffering in the world. When we heard that the Russians were coming, we had to hide my mother in the tool shed to prevent her from being raped. One day when my dad and I were on our way to the house to get food, we got caught in an air attack, and we had to run quickly back to the safety of the bunker. In the midst of the rapid machine gun fire, my father picked me up and carried me, running as fast as he could back to the bunker. We made it back alright; but the next day I saw with my own eyes the awful damage inflicted by the machine guns on the wall we had been running beside the day before. My mind travelled far away to the big world grandfather had told me about, where people were happy and peaceful.

When the war was over, we did our best to resume a normal life, but the Russian occupation was getting unbearable. At first it seemed like a good system, but it became progressively unbearable under the dictatorship of Stalin and the Hungarian statesmen Rakosi. Stalin was an autocrat, who made the village people fear to speak out at all against the Russians.

Even in the midst of hardship, though, there were happy times. Figure 2 shows one such occasion, in which my mother and I shared mutual happiness and laughter; Figure 3 shows the house where we lived; and Figure 4 is my Grandfather's family.

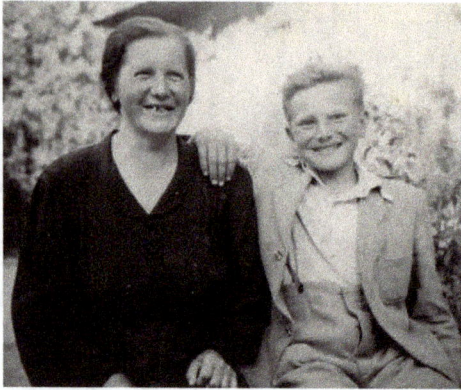

Figure 2: My mother and father and me

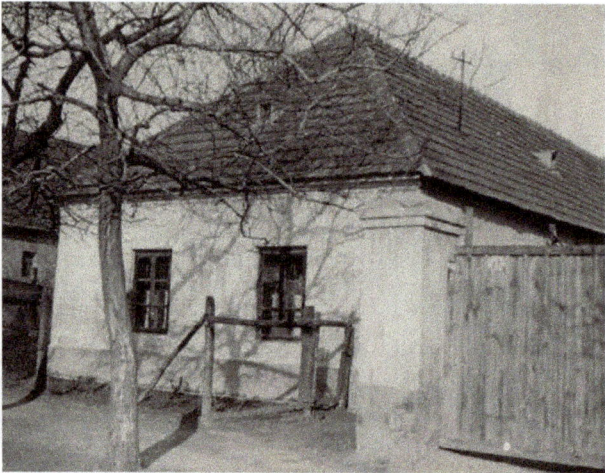

Figure 3: My family home

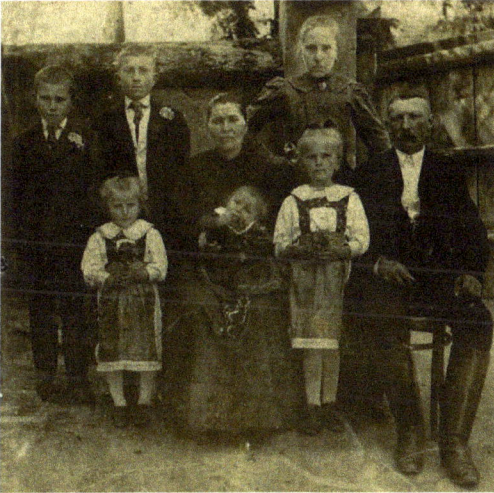

Figure 4: My Grandfather and his family

My father is on the right in the Picture; Grandfather and Grandmother had 6 children. As a young child, I would sit on grandfather's lap, as he told me his stories of the big world.

My father fought the communists and the system to the bitter end, until there was no produce left on the farm and we were forced into the collective farming system. By 1952 I had finished grade school, and I had to work in the forest to earn money for the family.

That winter my mother and I had to walk 3 miles on foot collecting acorns to sell as pig feed in order to earn enough money just to buy bread to eat. Once we had enough money, I had to go a full 10 Km to get to the bake shop to buy it. These were hard times, indeed.

When the opposition parties disbanded and the trade unions became ineffective, the churches became the main source of opposition to the communists. The government expropriated the churches' property in land reform; then, in July 1948, it nationalized church schools. Protestant church leaders reached a compromise with the government, but the head of the Roman Catholic Church, Cardinal Jozsef Mindszenty resisted. He was arrested on December 26, 1948. Rákosi, head of the communist party and Kádár, Minister of Interior, had determined that Mindszenty must confess, and Gábor Péter was told to extract a confession from him. They accused him of actively working against the democratic order of the Hungarian government, being a foreign spy, money laundering, and support of the fascists (even though he was jailed by the Arrow Party). He was also accused of trying to organize the Habsburgs to defeat the democratic government of the people. Of course Mindszenty denied these false accusations, and so the torture began. Mindszenty was taken to the headquarters of the AVH, located at 60 Andrássy ut, and forced into the unheated basement cellar (it was December 26th). AVH police mocked him as they tore off all his clothes. He was forced to change into a striped outfit, almost like something a clown would wear. The leader of the interrogation (AVH colonel) told him: "You better understand that the confession is not what you want to say but what we want to hear." Then the police wrote the confession and tried to force the Cardinal to sign. He refused, saying that the notes the police had taken of his confession were not his words. This angered the interrogators, so they began beating him with rubber batons. At which point another interrogator entered the room, ran at the Cardinal and began kicking him in the stomach with his heavy military boots. The beatings with the baton continued until the interrogators were exhausted. Yet, the Cardinal still refused to sign the "confession". The next day they showed him an article that was published in the national newspaper (Szabad Nép or Free Nation), which falsely reported that he had, in fact, confessed all his "sins". In spite of this, the torture continued; they still wanted him to actually sign the confession. AVH doctors came periodically to check on him and tried to force him to take medicine; he was afraid it might be drugs to confuse his mind, so he refused to swallow. The physical and mental torture continued for 39 days, until he was having difficulty recognizing reality. It was performed mainly at night, so as to afford him virtually no opportunity to sleep. Since he still refused to sign, the interrogators ended up forging his signature on a confession written by the head of AVH, General Gábor Péter, and the leader of the interrogation Colonel Décsi. On February 3rd, 1949 the doctors prepared the Cardinal for his "show trial," and on February 8th Rákosi's puppet judge Vilmos Olti sentenced Cardinal Mindszenty to life imprisonment.

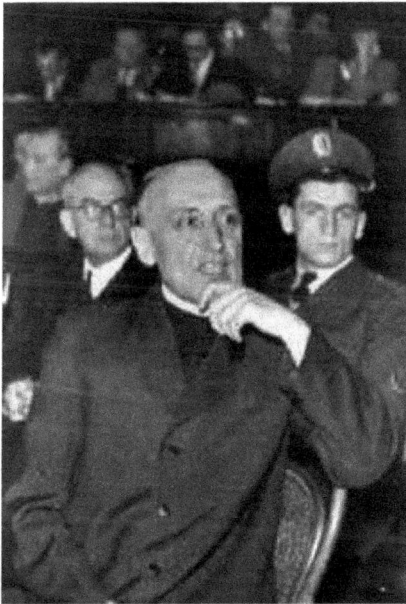

Figure 5. Mindszenty show trial. Rakosi is with glasses.

Totalitarian communism peaked during the period between 1949 and 1953. This was the darkest period in the history of Hungary, full of criminal activities and the sadistic control 3 top communist officials: Mátyás Rákosi (General Secretary of the Communist Party and after 1948 of the Hungarian Workers Party), Mihály Farkas (Minister of Defence) and Ernő Gerő (Deputy General Secretary of the Hungarian Workers party and Minister of Finance). The sadistic trio maintained their authoritarian dictatorship using fear tactics, imprisoning and executing leaders from the previous regime, high ranking communists who appeared to be a threat to the authority of the trio, religious leaders, and fellow communists who they framed with crimes that they themselves had committed. The latter occurred when Moscow called them to account for something they had done. While their crimes against humanity are many and varied, the following summary provides a general illustration of their total disregard for the law and the sanctity of human life. In 1950, under orders from Rákosi, the AVH established several forced labor or concentration camps for political prisoners. The most notorious of these camps was at Recsk in Heves County, Northern Hungary (Mátra Mountains) where 1,580 Hungarian citizens were interned for hard labor in the quarries. My Uncle was a prisoner in this camp. Rákosi's view was that political prisoners should not just be locked up, but also subjected to torture and hard labor, Soviet style. These prisoners were not given a trial; they were simply interned. Since these camps were so secretive, when prisoners were beaten to death, there was no accountability for their actions whatsoever at that time. Political prisoners were forced to work in the quarries, half-starved and frequently beaten by their jailers. Many prisoners died of exhaustion, in rock falls, or (more usually) while sleeping in muddy pits open to the sky. The cruelty of the AVH matched or even surpassed that of the SS and the KGB. The goal of the secret police was to protect the government, who they considered to be the communist party, and more specifically, its leaders who were then in control. My Uncle Istvan was imprisoned at Recsk for 5 years; he tried to cross the border to Yugoslavia, but the border guards turned him back to Hungary. He was finally freed when Nagy became prime minister.

During World War II, a communist cell headed by László Rajk, a veteran of the Spanish Civil War and a former student communist leader, operated underground within Hungary. Mátyás Rákosi led a second cell from Moscow. After the Soviet Red Army invaded Hungary in September 1944, Rajk's organization emerged from hiding and the Rákosi group returned to Hungary. Rákosi's close ties with the Soviets enhanced his influence within the party, and a rivalry developed between the Muscovites and Rajk's followers.

Rákosi described himself as "Stalin's best Hungarian disciple" and "Stalin's best pupil." He also invented the term "salami tactics," which referred to his approach of eliminating the opposition slice by slice.

In 1946 Rajk organized the Hungarian Communist Party's private army, the brutal secret police (AVH). Under the cover of "struggle against fascism and reaction" and "defense of the power of proletariat", he prohibited and liquidated several religious, national, democrat and maverick establishments and groups.

The communist infighting used anti-Titoism as an opportunity of getting rid of communists who favored national pride, some measure of independence, and especially those who were not trained in the Soviet Union. Rákosi saw Rajk as a threat to his power, so he decided to falsely accuse him of being an agent of Tito and had him arrested in 1949. Rákosi orchestrated Rajk's show trial mainly to please Stalin, who was furious with Tito. During the "show trial" Rajk was sentenced to death and later hanged.

Between the years of 1949 and 1952, Rákosi's regime practiced political cleansing, in which Hungarian families were deported to forced labor camps. There were 13 such camps, populated with 2,500 families totalling about 8,000 interns, which included able bodied men and women, as well as children and senior citizens. These deportations were not decided by any court of law, but simply at the whim of local communists and the political police. Rákosi imposed authoritarian rule and totalitarian communism on Hungary. During this time, an estimated 2,000 people were executed and over 100,000 were imprisoned. Some members of the Hungarian Workers Party opposed these policies, which led Rákosi, to expel them from the party.

In spite of all of this, in 1953, I was allowed to continue my education but had only been able to dream about the big world my grandfather had described. Then, in 1956 when the revolution started,

I signed on as a freedom fighter (at the time I was a 4th year high school student).

On the first day of the revolution I went home to the village, where I saw the uprising as it occurred. The village had a lot of turmoil, with much gossip from door to door, so the village priest suggested holding a Mass that evening. It was not formally announced, only the church bell sounded, inviting people to Mass. Dr. Lenarsics, the village priest, asked his assistants to ring the church bell at 5 o'clock, again at 5:15 pm and finally at 5:30 pm. By 5:30 pm, the church was packed with people all waiting for the village priest to make an announcement. The priest, however, said a Mass and during the homily he made an announcement in support of the uprising. He was passionate towards the revolution and suggested sending food to the students fighting in Budapest. Then after the Mass, he called upon someone to read the poem of Petöfi (it was composed at the 1848 revolution against Austria). I was just leaving the church when Dr. Lenarsics asked me to read it (I had recited this very poem during village celebrations in days gone by). So I began:

Talpra Magyar, hí a haza!
Itt az idő, most vagy soha!
Rabok legyünk vagy szabadok?
Ez a kérdés, válasszatok!
A magyarok istenére
Esküszünk,
Esküszünk, hogy rabok tovább
Nem leszünk!

Rabok voltunk mostanáig,
árhozottak ősapáink,
Kik szabadon éltek-haltak,
Szolgaföldben nem nyughatnak.
A magyarok istenére, Esküszünk,
Esküszünk, hogy rabok tovább,
Nem leszünk!

Sehonnai bitang ember,

Ki most, ha kell, halni nem mer,

Kinek drágább rongy élete,

Mint a haza becsülete.

A magyarok istenére, Esküszünk,

Esküszünk, hogy rabok tovább

Nem leszünk!

Fényesebb a láncnál a kard,

Jobban ékesíti a kart,

És mi mégis láncot hordtunk!

Ide veled, régi kardunk!

A magyarok istenére, Esküszünk,

Esküszünk, hogy rabok tovább

Nem leszünk!

A magyar név megint szép lesz,

Méltó régi nagy hiréhez;

Mit rákentek a századok,

Lemossuk a gyalázatot!

A magyarok istenére, Esküszünk,

Esküszünk, hogy rabok tovább

Nem leszünk!

Hol sírjaink domborulnak,

Unokáink leborulnak,

És áldó imádság mellett

Mondják el szent neveinket.

A magyarok istenére, Esküszünk,

Esküszünk, hogy rabok tovább

Nem leszünk!

It translates into English as follows:

On your feet, Magyar, the homeland calls!

The time is here, now or never!

Shall we be slaves or free?

This is the question, choose your answer! –

By the God of the Hungarians

We vow,

We vow, that we will be slaves
No longer!

We were slaves up until now,
Damned are our ancestors,
Who lived and died free,
Cannot rest in a slave land.
By the God of the Hungarians
We vow,
We vow, that we will be slaves
No longer

Useless villain of a man,
Who now, if need be, doesn't dare to die,
Who values his pathetic life greater
Than the honor of his homeland.
By the God of the Hungarians
We vow,
We vow, that we will be slaves
No longer!

The sword shines brighter than the chain,
Decorates better the arm,
And we still wore chains!
Return now, our old sword!
By the God of the Hungarians
We vow,
We vow, that we will be slaves
No longer!

The Magyar name will be great again,
Worthy of its old, great honor;
Which the centuries smeared on it,
We will wash away the shame!
By the God of the Hungarians
We vow,
We vow, that we will be slaves
No longer!

Where our grave mounds lie,
Our grandchildren will kneel,
And with blessing prayer,
Recite our sainted names.
By the God of the Hungarians
We vow,
We vow, that we will be slaves
No longer!

I recited the Hungarian national poem with full poetic flair, placing my hand over my chest, as I recited each verse. By the end of the poem, even my father was shouting the refrain:

By the God of the Hungarians
We vow,
We vow, that we will be slaves
No longer!

Well, the Hungarian national poem really excited the village people; from then on things occurred very rapidly, and I was elected leader of the Revolutionary Youth Council. By 10 pm, we were rounding up the local communists for trial. I convinced the council to try the communists when we return to power. In addition, we collected food supply, which we shipped to Budapest to aid the freedom fighters.

We won the revolution and the Russians began to pull out. The French and English, however, had invaded Egypt, which caused the Soviet government to take a second look at the situation, and the tanks rolled back into Hungary once again. The revolution was short lived, lasting only a few weeks before the Russian tanks rolled back in and ended the uprising. I was in a bind; my uncle had spent 5 years in Recsk a political prisoner, and I was certain I would be captured and executed. As the Russians rounded up the freedom fighters, imprisoning and killing them, I made my escape to Austria. I was 18 years old at the time and spoke only Hungarian. But now my dream of seeing the "big world" was becoming a reality. It was, however, quite different from the one my grandfather had described. We were subjected to policemen, who curtailed our freedom; we were unable to even leave the compound.

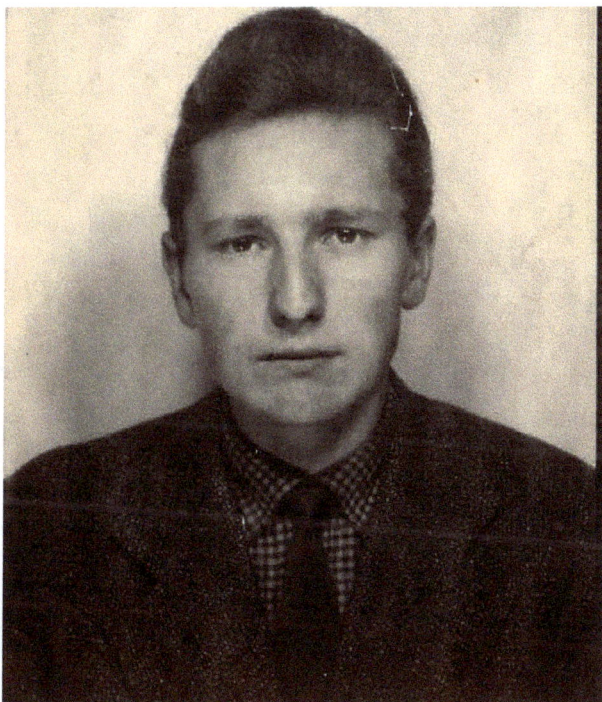

Figure 6. First picture as I escaped from Hungary.

however, made a return from the rear of the house.
Not once did Wilson suspect the policeman was
outside. Soon, Jackson was under arrest, sitting in
the back of

Photograph of a picture to keep up compromising

THE BIG WORLD

Soldiers came to guard the refugee camps after a few weeks, and we were effectively cut off from the outside world. So, I joined a group of refugees destined for England. We took a train near Graz bound for Salzburg. The kindness of strangers and their basket of apples sustained us on the train, as we had brought nothing to eat; but, by the time we got to Salzburg, we were really quite hungry. There we were met by the Red Cross, who gave us cheese and cradle. I was so famished I positively devoured the food, but had to fly to London in less than an hour, which I found concerning. In case of sickness brought on by exhaustion, the excitement of my first flight, and rapid ingestion of food, I sat on the plane with a handkerchief over my mouth. Thankfully, I was okay.

After landing in, we were taken to an army barracks in Aldershot, where we served as interns. We were surrounded by gates guarded by soldiers, so once again I found myself in a locked compound.

Soldiers and government officials interviewed the interns to weed out potential spies trying to escape to the west. I saw some people disappear during this time, but most remained. After about a week, 10 of us were transported to Halifax, Yorkshire, where we stayed in the Salvation Army hostel for about one week more; the hostel smelled a bit, but the food was quite good. Then, finally, we were able to rent a cottage and have real accommodations of our own. An English lady, Mrs. Dillinger, became our interpreter and assisted us in the transition to a new country. After Christmas I was able to obtain a job processing trousers in a textile factory. My cousin Imre and another refugee Zoltan joined me there in the same line of work. And so began my life in at new country. We found the locals friendly and helpful; we felt welcomed and accepted.

Our rental cottage was on the outskirts of Halifax, leading to Hebden Bridge, where we worked. I did my best to pick up English from the factory workers, who had a distinctive Yorkshire accent. Fortunately it came easy to me, and I progressed quite rapidly. A young office lady who worked in the factory helped me a lot with my English. I also attended a local church on Sundays, where I met a nice family, Mr. and Mrs. Gillespie, who helped me to adjust to my new life. Their two daughters, Maureen and Kathleen (slightly my senior) took me around town and introduced me to fellow high school students. This was wonderful, and Mr. and Mrs. Gillespie treated me just like a son. While the other refugees were spending the night in pubs, I went a different route, choosing rather to pursue intellectual interests and learn English. I told Mrs. Gillespie that I had been a high school student when the revolution broke out, and I was anxious to continue my studies. And then one day after work, I discovered that Mrs. Gillespie had met with the local high school principal to discuss options for furthering my education. Because my English was still pretty rudimentary, I chose to take entrance exams pertaining to mathematics. I passed the test at a first-year university level, thankful now that I had majored in math my final year in high school. Mrs. Gillespie then informed me of the opportunity to attend university as a final year high school student. We discussed which major I ought to pursue. In Hungary I had been admitted to law school, but in Britain I decided on a different course of study altogether. I would take a science track and study forestry. This course of study gave me the opportunity to work outdoors for a year in the bush, and I felt it was the best option available.

Mrs. Gillespie assisted me in my college search, and soon I was accepted in Edinburgh, Scotland. In order to matriculate, I had to pass a final exam in English and covering the subjects of zoology, chemistry, botany, and physics. I passed, but only earned wages equal to that of the factory work I had done.

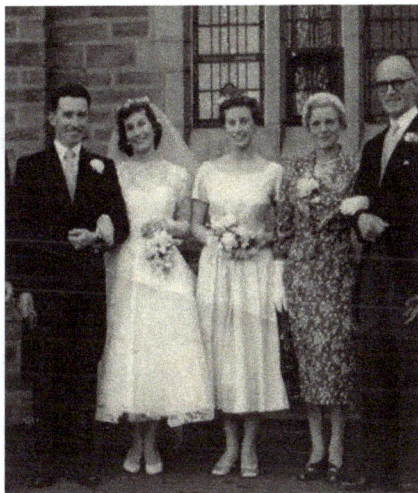

Figure 8: Mr. and Mrs. Gillespie and family

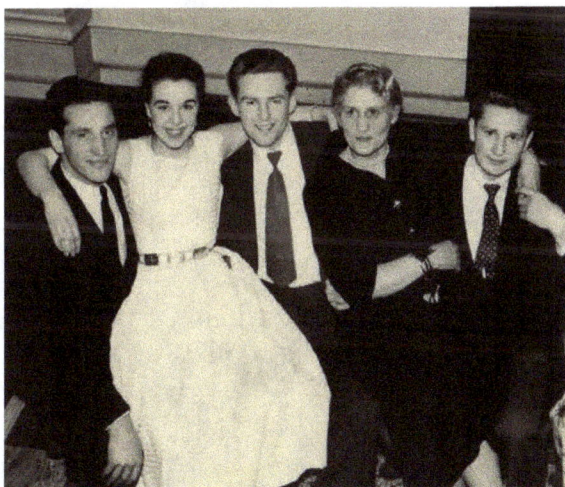

Figure 9: Mrs. Dillinger and I with Zoltan (far left).

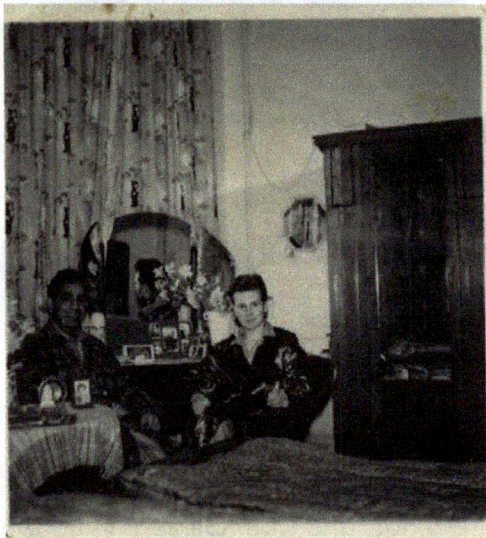

Figure 10: First year at University.

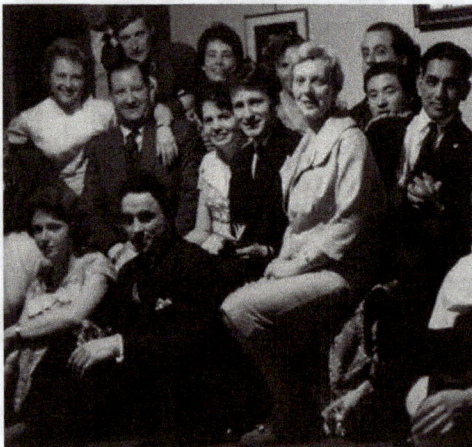

Figure 11: My 21st birthday party.

After four years of study in Edinburgh, I graduated with a degree in Forestry. During my 3rd year I got married; and about a year later, my wife and I had a son. The story my grandfather had always told me about the "big-world" seemed to actually be coming true. I was finally living it.

STARTING OF A NEW LIFE

After graduating, I worked for three years as an explorer in the Amazon Rain Forest. I found it very interesting, and was even able to spend three months out of each year actually working in the jungle. I was there during the time; British Guiana was fighting for its independence.

The job began with my arrival in Georgetown on Tuesday. December 4th 1961; there I was met by Mr. Jeffrey Phillips, the Deputy Conservator of Forests, who took me to a guest house on Murray Street. Thankfully it was within walking distance of the Forestry Department office on Kingston Road, as I had no money to buy a car. At 8 a.m., the very next morning, I went to the office and reported to Mr. Dow, the Conservator of Forests. The moment I saw him I recognized him: He was the man I had met in London who had asked me if I wanted to work in South America. He greeted me with a big smile and I immediately felt very comfortable about my first professional job. Mr. Dow did an excellent job on my orientation. He informed me that Mr. Tom Reese, who was also part of the interview panel, would be arriving shortly to train me on leading expeditions in the jungle. By February 1st 1962, my coworkers had helped arrange my rental of a furnished house in Georgetown. Mr. Phillips even offered to help me hire domestic help; but, I said I was fine without it. He said that hiring domestic help would aid the local economy, so we hired an Amerindian woman named Lena for BG$ 30 per month plus room and board. She had a 3 year old daughter, named Lisa. Lena was happy to have the opportunity to work for us and stayed the entire three years. Yet these were turbulent political times in British Guiana. The governing party was the Peoples Progressive Party (PPP), led by Dr. Cheddi Jagan, a US educated dentist of East Indian descent. The main opposition party was the Peoples National Congress (PNC), led by Forbes Burnham, representing the people of African descent. The other opposition party was the United Force (UF), led by Peter D'Aguiar of Portuguese descent, standing for big business interests. D'Aguiar owned the brewery, was connected to the right wing religious groups, and controlled the local paper, called the Chronicle. Although Dr. Jagan had won a democratic election in 1961, the opposition was not willing to accept the results in spite of the majority vote. Dr. Jagan was also considered a communist, which opened him up to attack from several sources, with D'Aguiar at the forefront. And, during the 1961 election, the Christian Social Council openly campaigned against the PPP.

My wife and son arrived in Georgetown on February 14th 1962; it was the first time I would see my son, so I was very excited. Immediately after disembarking, Audrey handed Michael, who had been named after my grandfather, over to me. We picked up the luggage and headed to our rental house in the Forestry Department. Audrey was surprised to find that we had domestic help; but after hearing the explanation and tasting the great meal Lena had prepared for dinner, she seemed quite pleased..

The next day, Mr. Phillips drove us around Georgetown, where we walked along the famous sea wall. Audrey and I were excited about living in the tropics, enjoying the palm trees, and experiencing the warm climate with its tropical showers. In the mist of our tropical paradise, however, a dismal political cloud loomed overhead; and, we felt nervous at the escalating disturbances.

My wife and I watched from the balcony of rental house as looters robbed furniture and other items from the local residents. This was a new experience for us, and we began to have second thoughts, especially as we considered the safety of our young son. After a few days, though, the city got back to "normal," and we gradually adjusted to our new environment. Michael, in particular, seemed to enjoy the tropical climate.

That March Mr. Tom Reese, from the Department of Technical Cooperation in London, arrived to train me to lead expeditions in the jungle. He was the former Conservator of Forests in Nigeria, and a very kind Englishman, who observed tradition in a rather original manner. He was there for 3 months and trained me at the office in aerial photo interpretation, and, as promised, provided training in the bush. To avoid the rainy season which lasted from mid-May to mid-August, my jungle training was conducted in April in the Bartica Triangle. Prior to going out on the expedition, I asked Mr. Reese for advice on what to wear. He told me what type of boots to get, as well as the clothing, including a dressing gown. Mr. Reese insisted on wearing a dressing gown while away from home, which I thought was an unusual custom. The first day in the jungle with Mr. Reese was quite memorable. Our camp consisted of a tarpaulin top, a ground sheet, two camp cots with mosquito netting, and one folding table with two chairs. We woke at 6 am, put on our dressing gowns, and sat down, while the camp attendant served us coffee. After that we went down to the creek, where we discarded our dressing gowns and pyjamas and bathed in the nude. The dressing gown custom, however, was taken a step further, as we put them on again when we returned to the camp to eat breakfast. After breakfast Romalho, the camp attendant, walked by and shouted "paper?" to which Mr. Reese, after steadily fixing his eyes on him, responded "Yes.". Romalho brought the air edition of The Times to Mr. Reese and was paid 25 cents. Romalho had a total of 20 newspapers, which Mr. Reese read consecutively, one per day, starting with the oldest first. When Mr. Reese saw the puzzlement on my face, he explained that in order to keep your sanity in the jungle, it helps to recreate as much of your home environment as possible, hence the dressing gowns and morning newspaper.

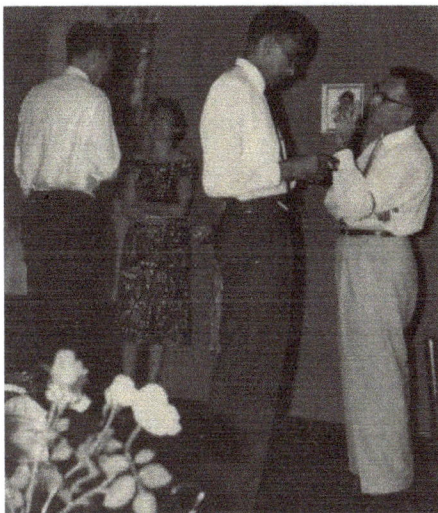

Figure 12: From r to l: Mr. Reese, Dow and Philips

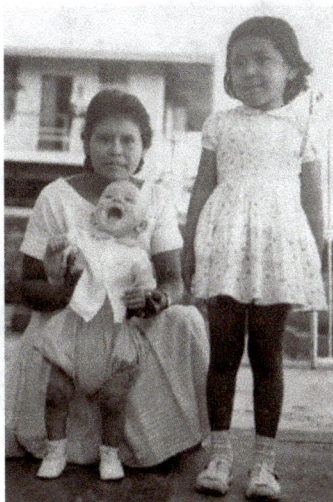

Figure 13: Our domestic help Lena, Michael and Lisa

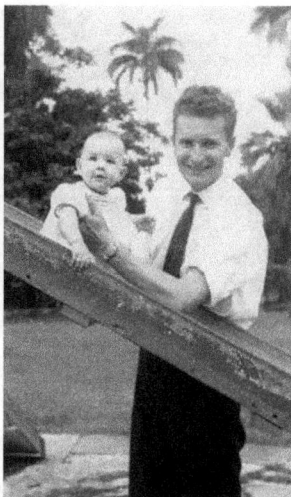

Figure 14: Myself with Michael

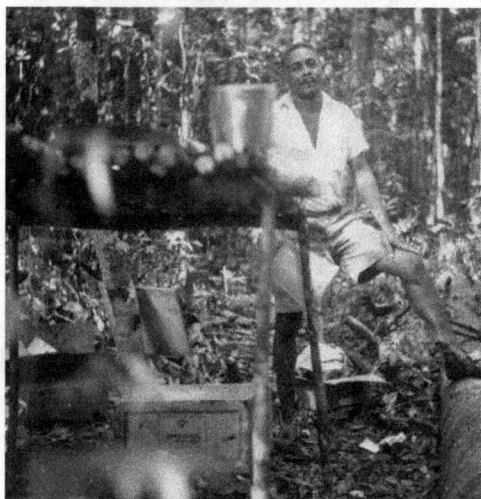

Figure 15: Romalho, the kitchen chief

I passed Mr. Reese's training session and organized my first expedition for mid-August to mid-November, the next dry season. We targeted an area along the Cuyuni River where some good greenheart timber stands (*Ocotea rodiaei* of the family Lauraceae) had been spotted from the air. This area, which had never been surveyed before, was not accessible by road. An air survey company obtained aerial photographs at a scale of 1:15,000 but I had no base maps with which to compare them, so I had to obtain ground control information as part of the expedition. First, I interpreted the aerial photos in stereo, creating polygons of homogeneous strata. The idea was to obtain a more accurate and precise description of the polygons after identifying trees and forest types on the ground during the survey. Using the photographs, I planned the camp sites and the survey lines, and then flew over the area, with a local tree spotter, on a single engine Cessna aircraft. The pilot was an experienced bush pilot, who loved aerobatics. I remember looking down to see the trees and suddenly being met with a view of the sky as he flew the plane upside down. When he straightened out, I asked him to descend a little so we could identify tree species. At which point he took me down so far that I could almost touch their leaves. It took two and a half hours to collect the necessary information; and by the time we landed, both the tree spotter and I looked rather pale, which delighted the pilot. After the visual reconnaissance, I started planning the ground expedition. The first task was to recruit 45 experienced men to work in the jungle. I did the recruiting from within the town of Bartica; and, within a week, managed to get a good team together. Rufus Boyan, an Amerindian and Inspector in the Forestry Department, was my technical lead and right hand man. He had been trained by a famous English botanist, Mr. Fanshawe, and knew the names of over 200 tree species in both English and Latin. Oscar Sampson, a Forest Ranger of African origin, managed the team of men on the expedition. Capt. Wong was in charge of the 16-foot cabin cruiser and his job was to make sure we reach the survey site, carefully steering us up the treacherous Mazaruni and Cuyuni Rivers. We started out from Bartica and entered the mouth of the Mazaruni River at Essequibo, and then up the challenging Cuyuni. The cabin cruiser was followed by 6 boats with outboard motors, and on the Cuyuni we often had to pull the boats up over the fast flowing rapids. This was quite an experience. It took eight men on each bank to do the job, each pulling hard on the ropes attached to the boats. The Captain asked me to go ashore and walk along, but I chose to stay with him instead. Capt. Wong was very experienced and in full command of the situation, as he directed the men pulling the boats over the steep rapids. We had a few close calls when the men slipped back rather than going forward; but after two gruelling hours the ordeal was over. We had now reached a higher level of the Cuyuni River which, thankfully, was flat. After the cabin cruiser was in safe waters, the crew went behind and pulled each of the other six boats following us to safety. We then traveled several more hours on the Cuyuni until we reached the site I had spotted from the air during visual reconnaissance.

On the shore of the Cuyuni River, we built a temporary base camp. My camp, however, was built further back from the shore of the Cuyuni, up a small creek, so that I would always have clean water to drink. All tents consisted of tarpaulin set atop an A frame, with no sides, and a ground sheet. My tent had the addition of mosquito netting hanging from the top beam, and inside was a camp cot, a folding table with two chairs, and an oil lantern. Romalho kept the supply tent about 30 yards down the creek. The remaining crew found accommodations in 5 tents further down the creek, about 200 yards from Romalho's. They slept in hammocks, about 8-10 hanging under each tarpaulin tent. We had supplies in sufficient quantity to last us three months. The crew supplies consisted of salt fish, salt beef, rice and tea. In my supplies were the addition of canned vegetables and one bottle of Demerara rum for each week of the expedition. Under my control, we also carried 4 shotguns (16 gauge double barrels) for general use, several cases of ammunition, one large case of medicine, 12 lanterns, several cans of fuel, and pots and pans for each tent. The medicine kit supplied by a government chemist in Georgetown included 8 boxes of anti-snake bite, which required refrigeration. When I realized this back in Georgetown, I asked Rufus Boyan what the Amerindians use against snake bites. He said they used a native mixture made from different plants that was called Especifico; upon receiving this information we added 8 bottles of Especifico to the medicine kit.

We headed out from the base camp, cutting a compass line 5 miles in a northerly direction. The bush was very thick; the natives called it ropey forest.

The compass man had to be followed by two line cutters, who cleared a path for the crew carrying the supplies. Next in line came two chain-men, who measured the distance one chain (66 feet) at a time, marking the distance with a wooden peg at each chain length. When the crew reached the 5 mile mark, we pegged the location of the base camp, with my camp again being higher up on the creek. The crew then dismantled the temporary base camp, moving all tents to the new location, except one that was left for Capt. Wong and his crew. All of this had to be completed in one day, so that we could settle into our new base camp before dark. Crew members carried the supplies and tents on their backs in a long basket strapped on their shoulders, and supported by another strap on their forehead. A fit person could carry 80-105 pounds five miles without a problem. As we walked up the line, my body guard cautioned me to be alert, especially where snakes were concerned. Labaria (*Lachesis lanceolatus*), an exceedingly poisonous snake, was our biggest concern. It is rarely more than four feet in length; but, its bite, if not treated properly, can be fatal within 48 hours. I quickly learned how to spot these snakes because, each day, at least one of them would try to bite me. I always walked with a long stick I could use to kill them. When attacked by a larger snake such as the Bushmaster, (*Lachesis muta muta),* I had to make the kill with a shotgun. The Bushmaster is a huge, thick-bodied and highly venomous snake; it has a triangularly shaped head, one of nature's warning signs that a snake is poisonous and potentially deadly. The first one of these cruel dudes (as they were coined by the natives) I met was about 10 feet long. It struck at me on a trail, going for my upper body. The Bushmaster is capable of multiple bite strikes, injecting large amounts of venom; even the bite of a juvenile Bushmaster can be fatal. I always walked with a loaded shotgun and managed to shoot the snake with its head barely a few feet from me. There was no time for hesitation; one had to act quickly and decisively. I was told that on average, almost half of the leaders in an expedition like mine, would either die of snake bite, insect bite, or animal attack; they might even be killed by their crew. These odds were pretty sobering. Our second day at the base camp was spent cleaning up and making everyone comfortable. Two men spent most of the day building a toilet for me; it consisted of two pieces of wood (5 inches X 3 feet) dug into the ground 4 feet apart. It was   2 feet above ground, with a V branch at the upper end. They even made a toilet seat for me using a 6 foot long, smooth, straight piece of wood (5 inches in diameter). It was placed on the V ends of the vertical poles to make the seat. Under the seat, was a deep hole, which completed the design of my outdoor toilet. Mr Reese taught me an important aspect of my duty as expedition leader was to be decisive and in full control at all times. This was not for ego, but to make the crew feel comfortable under guidance of a strong leader. To that end, each morning Sampson lined up the crew single file, and I addressed each person by name and gave him his assignment. These instructions involved which survey line and task they were assigned, such as marking the line with a compass, cutting the path behind the compass man, measuring the distance with the chain, identifying a type of tree and measuring its diameter at breast height with a calliper, hunting for meat, and being my personal body guard for the day. After tasting the salt fish and beef, I decided to designate a hunter to get fresh meat for the crew each day. Romalho told me that this was the best morale builder he had seen in all his years in the jungle. The crew enjoyed having fresh meat almost every day; and when it could not be obtained they always had the dry salt fish and beef available. I rotated the body guard, who walked beside me to protect me from natural hazards, as this was considered to be a cushy job. The position was used as a reward for good work by crew members. This way I also got to know my crew members individually and bonded with those who responded to the challenge. I was in top physical condition and could walk 15-20 miles each day under rugged terrain, which earned me considerable respect from the crew.

The three months we spent surveying the timber supply of the Cuyuni River area were really eventful. There were no sign that that area had ever been settled by humans. Yet, when we were digging up the ground to build our base camp, I found a stone carving of a powis (bush turkey) head. On the expedition, I also learned to appreciate what Mr. Reese had taught me about jungle survival. After two months out there, it became important to distinguish one week from another. So on Sundays, I would dress up in my Sunday best: Dress pants, white short sleeved shirt, and black leather shoes. I ate my lunch with a glass of juice, after which I would invite Romalho to have a glass of rum with me.

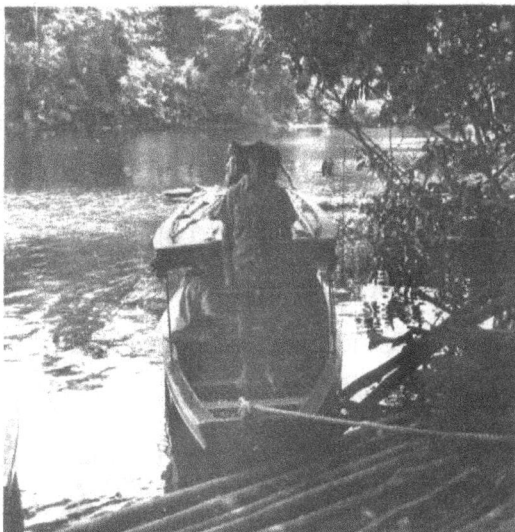

Figure 16: Captain Wong and a cabin cruiser.

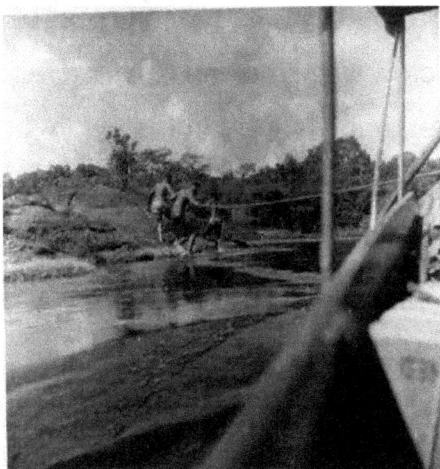

Figure 17: The Cabin cruiser in the rapids.

By 1963 I had taken several trips to the Bartica Savannah. The roads were generally single lane, so if you were unfortunate enough to meet a logging truck coming from the opposite direction, fully loaded with timber that would not be able to stop in time, the only option was to get off the road and into the bush, provided you were not blocked by a large tree.

My second major expedition was conducted in the North West District, close to the Venezuelan border. We left Georgetown on Monday, August 19, 1963 at 1:50 pm on a ship called Steamer and arrived in Mabaruma the next day. I took most of the Cuyuni expedition crew with me, and we recruited about a dozen more men in Mabaruma, who had detailed knowledge of the region. We were to survey an area near the Venezuelan border during a time in which the border dispute between Venezuela and British Guiana had reached its peak. Hence, we carried more shotguns than we did during the Cuyuni expedition. Just prior to the expedition, we were visited by several high ranking government officials, including Mr. Brindley Benn, Minister of Natural Resources. We then headed out, with our boats traveling up the Wayne River to the site that I had earlier identified as our first base camp entrance during aerial reconnaissance. During the expedition, I was in the cabin cruiser with Capt. Wong and several of the senior staff. The rest of the men followed us in boats fitted with outboard motors. We traveled at night and the men started to sing "Old Man River;" the natives began waving at us from the river banks with lit torches in their hands. Even a Hollywood movie couldn't have made this scene more exciting or romantic. In the morning, we arrived at our destination tied up the boats on the river bank, and prepared to cut a straight line to the first base camp. Then, Rufus Boyan noticed some movements in the bush; we wondered what it could be. It did not sound like wild animals, and we were certain that there was no human settlement around there. So, I sent out a small group of Amerindian men to scout the area. In a couple of hours they returned with a native man, who spoke only the local dialect and had never before seen a white man. In fact, the tribe to which he belonged lived in total isolation from the rest of the Amerindians. Rufus Boyan managed to convince him that our expedition was a peaceful one, and I was invited to meet with the village elders under a thatch-roofed hut. We sat around in a circle, sharing a peace pipe, and the natives offered us their version of wine, which I agreed to sample, but found it tasted like vinegar. Rufus interpreted as I explained the details of the expedition. The elders then gave me permission to travel through the area to the base camp site. That night I slept on the boat, while the men slept in their hammocks hung from trees near the river bank. The next morning we started out early, cutting the line to the base camp site and transporting the supplies. We completed the task by early afternoon and had time to build the camp. My tent was, as usual, up river, with my camp attendant Romalho about 100 feet downstream with the kitchen and supplies. The rest of the crew put up their tents about 100 feet further down the creek. I went to bed at about 11 pm and slept well on my camp cot under the mosquito netting. But, at around 5 a.m., I woke to the sound of female laughter. This was unbelievable in the jungle. As I opened my eyes, I saw about half a dozen young Amerindian girls, 18-20 years old, looking down at me and giggling. They were barely covered with their breasts totally exposed as they bent down to examine me more closely. I lay thinking, "I've died and gone to heaven," and I was quite content to stay there. This moment of ecstasy, however, was short lived, and I soon heard the sound of my crew laughing as they asked me to get up and change. I got out of my camp cot and asked Rufus to tell the young ladies to go back to their village. Apparently, the village elders had told the girls of this pale-faced man, and they had decided to come to see it for themselves. They were not responding to Rufus' request, and I was just stood there waiting for the opportunity to get dressed. It wasn't happening, and the crew was enjoying my predicament, as they waited for me to give them their daily assignments. So, I decided to shave. I used a small mirror hung on a tree beside a wooden table with a water basin.   I poured some water into the basin and looked into the mirror. I could see the girls looking into the mirror with fascination. They had had no contact with the outside world; and, seeing themselves in the mirror was very different than seeing their reflection in a clear bowl of water or the creek. I used the opportunity to divert their attention from me, and I handed them the mirror and went to the other side of the tent to change. Soon after, the girls left, and I was able to line up the crew for another day's work.

On November 3rd, we completed the North West District expedition, and the anticipated Venezuelan attack never materialized, for which I was very grateful. After returning to Georgetown, we did, however, experienced civil disobedience that was often life threatening. I sat with a loaded gun beside the window at night, and soon after that, sent the family back to Edinburgh. I also sold my car and bought a motorcycle instead for transportation.

On Monday, August 31st, 1964, I started my third and final expedition in the Bartica Triangle. This time, the expedition site was accessible by Land Rovers. However, by this time, racial tensions had escalated in different parts of the country. This worried me because my crew consisted of people of African, Indian, Portuguese and Amerindian descent. I met with the crew at our base camp and had a dialogue with them which re-established my faith in the human race. I asked the men to "look at each other with tolerance and mutual respect. Let's survive the elements of the jungle together. We are all brothers and not each other's enemy." The crew responded well, and after that, we just focused on getting the job done and looking after each other.

The Bartica Triangle expedition also turned out to be quite eventful. Even though a single dirt lane road provided us access to the area, danger was still present with us. One day as I was walking on a narrow trail, I was suddenly confronted by a 10-foot-long bushmaster. Fortunately, I had sensed the danger, so both my body guard and I were equipped with loaded shotguns. As the bushmaster struck at me, his head about 4 feet of the ground, I managed to shoot him in the head, and the snake then dropped about 2 feet away from me. My body guard Banjee yelled out with excitement "you got it just in time chief!" I acted relatively cool; but when we got back to the camp, I said to Romalho: "it is time to have a glass of rum". He rushed the rum to my tent and stood there nervously, wanting to know what had happened. He knew that I only drank rum during the day when something really scary happened. A few days later

Romalho cautioned me to be careful at night because he had been sensing movement around the camp. He thought it might be a wild hog or even a jaguarondi. I went to bed around midnight, turned down the lantern a little bit and kept my loaded shotgun besides me; just as I started to drift off, I sensed something approaching my tent. In a flash, I saw a jaguarondi lunging towards me. I had just enough time to roll to the side and fire the gun wildly. The jaguarondi hit the camp cot, which was now on my back, and ran off into the dark, scared by the sound of gunfire. Romalho ran over to see what had happened; I was pretty shaken; he just looked at me and said: "I'll bring the rum, sir." After that, we stayed up the rest of the night just in case the cat decided to come back.

Near the end of the expedition, a British Army Officer, Lt. John Foster visited me at my base camp. He had a camp in the Bartica Triangle about 5 miles from where I was. His camp was set up in the former residence of the regional manager of BG Timbers lumber company. His camp was outfitted with a fridge, stove, and even indoor plumbing, which was a great luxury at that time in the bush. Our expedition was completed in early November.

When I got back to Georgetown, I finished my report and began packing my belongings. My wife and son were already in Edinburgh, Scotland, staying with her parents. As part of my contract, I was given 6 months paid leave and a trip back to Scotland. Mr. Dow said that he would be happy to have me for another 3 year contract; he suggested that I think it over and let him know in a couple of months. On December 1st, I shipped my stuff (we had no furniture, just clothes) back to Edinburgh and moved into the Tower Hotel, while waiting for a fight out. Getting out of Georgetown was not easy; a general strike had shut down all of Atkinson Airport. On December 2nd, some friends invited me to a party where I met some Canadians from the High Commission. They suggested that I visit Toronto on my way back to Scotland because Canada was looking for people with college degrees in forestry. The next day I went to the Canadian High Commission and obtained a 10-day-visitor's-visa to travel through Canada. By this time, I was on standby, waiting for a flight to get out. On December 4th, while having a drink in the bar, Miss. DeFreitas, a former neighbor, stopped by to say hello. She was an airline hostess with Air France, and I asked her to help me get to Trinidad. She said that she was flying to Trinidad the next day with some people who the strikers had allowed out. She suggested that I travel with her to the airport, in order to get past the picketers. So, on December 5th I got behind Miss DeFreitas on her scooter, with my small suitcase in between us, and headed to the airport. She was wearing her uniform, so we were able to get through the picket line. I already had my full-fare airline ticket from British Airways, which was accepted for only the portion of the flight from Georgetown to Port of Spain.

Realizing it would be complicated to sort out my travel plans, I checked into a hotel next to the airport, and then headed back inside to sort out the flight. I took my full-fare ticket from British Airways to Air Canada and asked them if I could use it to fly to Scotland via Toronto. They were happy to accept it, and gave me a new ticket that allowed me to visit both Toronto and Montreal before going back to Glasgow.

IMMIGRATED TO CANADA

In Canada I applied for jobs in the Ontario Government and was offered a position with Ontario Lands and Forests. So, we immigrated to Canada. Our daughter Jennifer was soon born in Toronto, Canada; now we were blessed with two children, a boy and a girl!

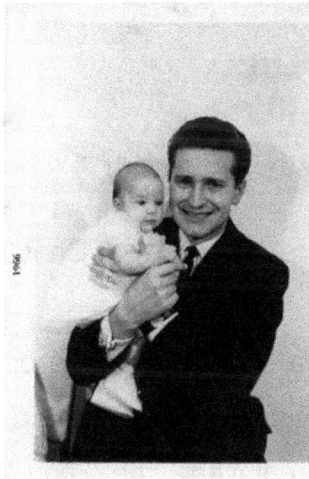

Figure 18: I am holding Jennifer

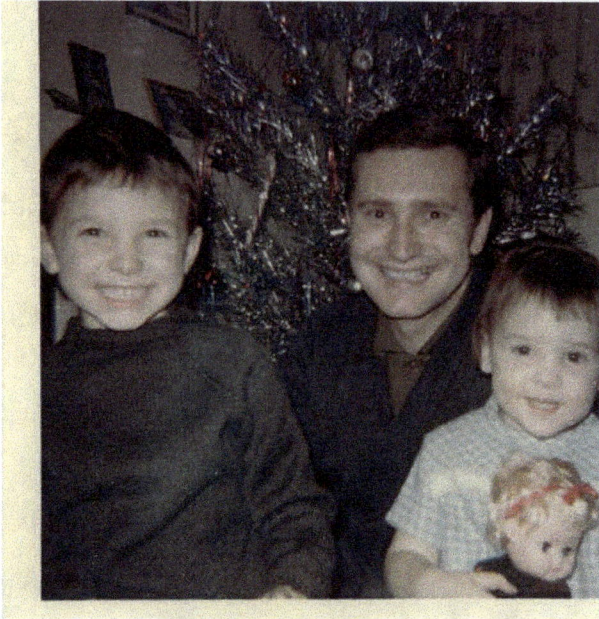

Figure 19: Happy at Christmas

In Canada, I decided to go back to school to get a M.Sc. Degree in statistics, mensuration and silviculture. I enjoyed the courses, especially mensuration and silviculture. The statistics part was mostly lectures exams. However, I got a good mark in all subjects, and now I was ready to tackle my doctorate. I was accepted at the University of British

Columbia to study modelling. My Master's program was covered by the government (50 % funding) plus fees, and I was offered the same funding for my doctorate. Shortly after my decision to study for my doctorate, my wife decided to leave me and our children. Here is was with a broken marriage and two children to rise on my own, my daughter being only 3-years-old at the time. I got in touch with my Director and turned down the doctorate program. Then, my parents came over from Hungary to help me to look after the children. I raised the family as a single parent for a year, and after that I married a woman named Rose, who had a five-year-old son. We were married on June 30th, 1970. Rose used to tease me about the business manner in which I shopped at stores; I just made a bee line for the merchandise I wanted, and then headed straight home. She preferred to leisurely peruse the merchandise, looking around as she shopped; but, I was there to just get the job done and go home.

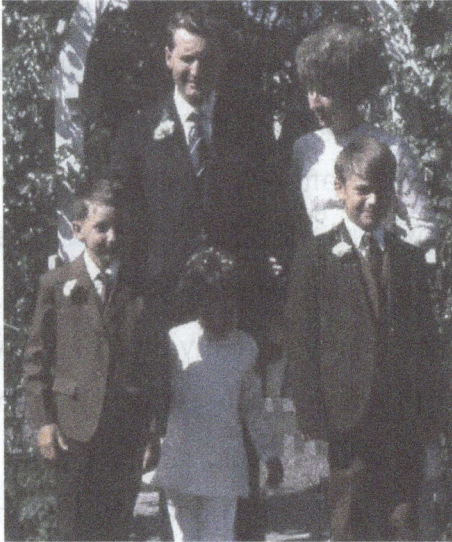

Figure 20: My marriage with Rose

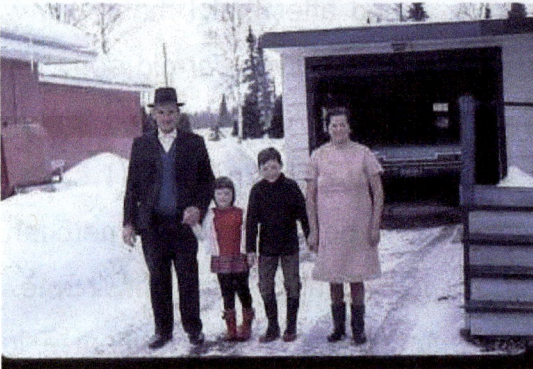

Figure 21: My parents helping to look after my
children

My career was very successful, and I held a few different positions in Victoria. Later, I started coaching hockey and spending time horseback riding with Jennifer.

.

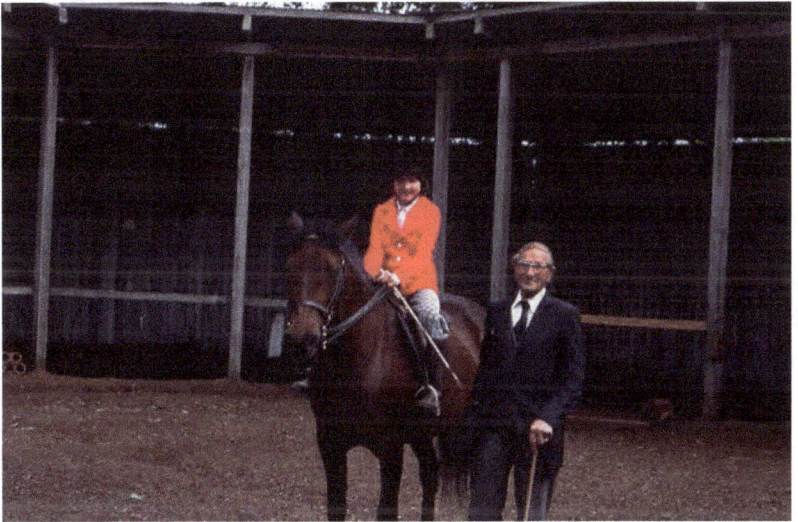

Figure 22: Jennifer riding with Mr. Carley

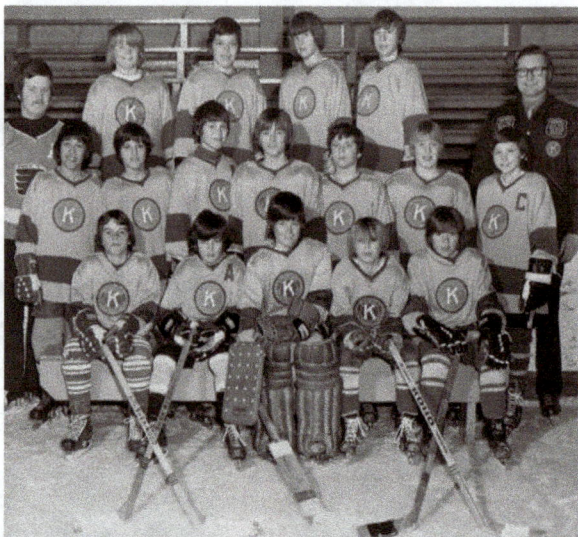

Figure 23: I coached the Kiwanis team (Michael wearing C)

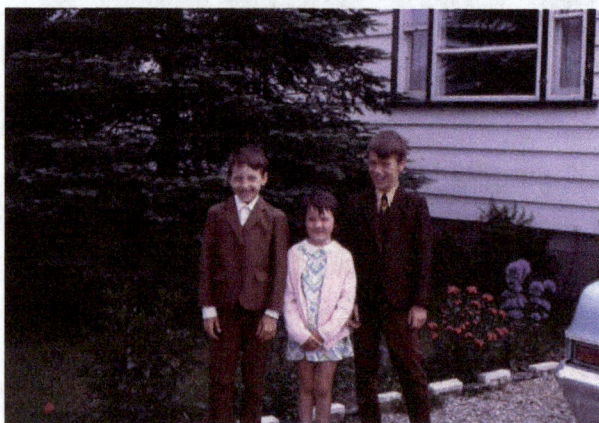

Figure 24: The blended family

In June 1974, 18 years after I had left, we returned to Hungary and visited with my family. When I had left Hungary I was only 18 years old, and there I was back there again 18 years later with two University degrees to my name. My grandfather was correct about a happier world in a far-away land.

In 1974 the Hungarian government was still communist, and I had to watch what I said. In Canada, I was a research scientist just beginning to publish my work. While I Hungary, I realized that researchers there had been exposed to my work, even studies I had not thought would reach them. We visited a few of research stations in Hungary, and received an excellent reception, which was great. The four weeks flew by, though, and before we knew it we had to get back to Canada.

My career was very professionally successful and I travelled to the world promoting Geographic Information Systems. In 1982, I even visited The Soviet Union as part of a scientific exchange. We travelled to Moscow, Leningrad and Kiev; the Soviet officials treated us well. In October 1985 I visited China to make a presentation on the peaceful use of outer space technology in resource management. In 1988, I was attended a conference on ISPRS and received the honor of being elected chairman of Commission VII. For four years I travelled everywhere promoting the environment and organizing workshops.

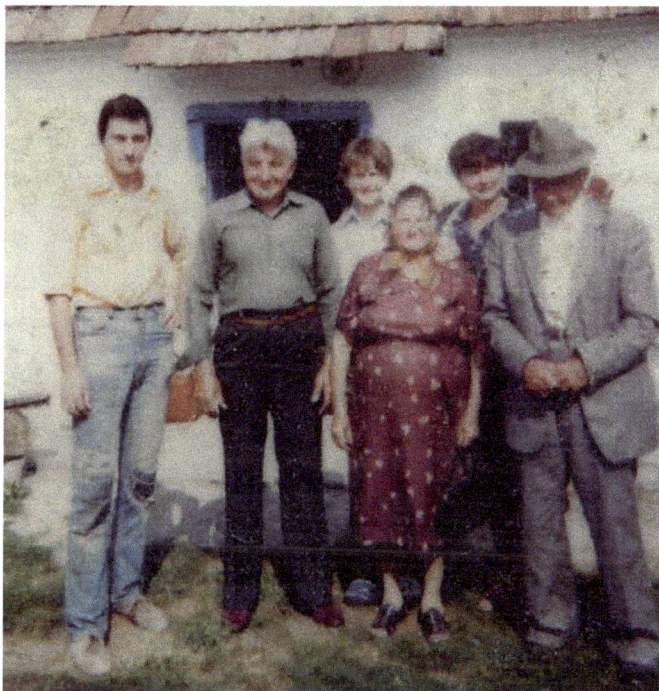

Figure 25: My Uncle (white haired) after he spent 5 years at Recsk as a political prisoner

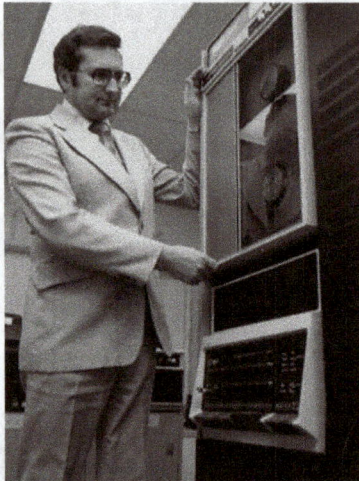

Figure 26: A most advanced computer graphics system in 1980

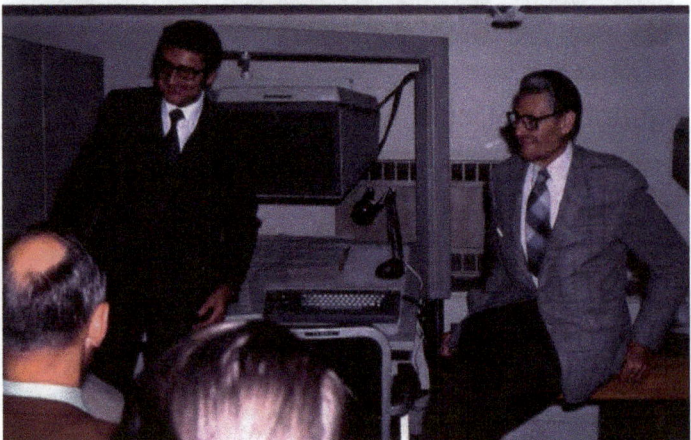

Figure 27: Computer graphics station

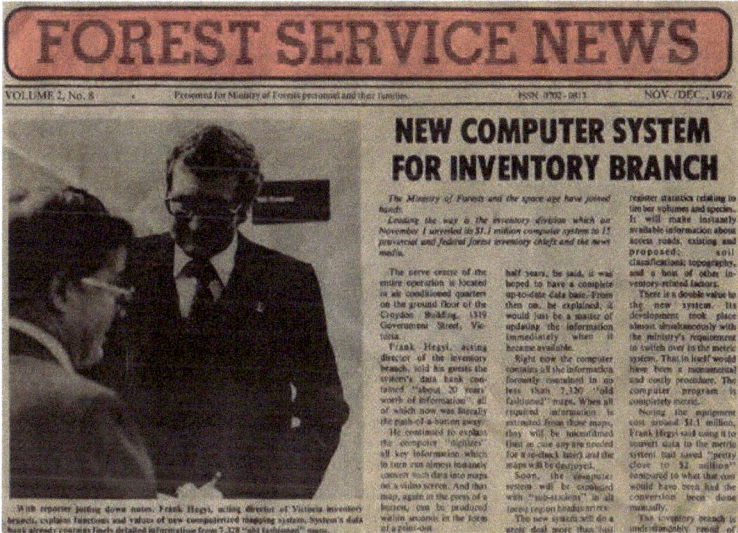

Figure 28: I was interviewed on TV for the computer system

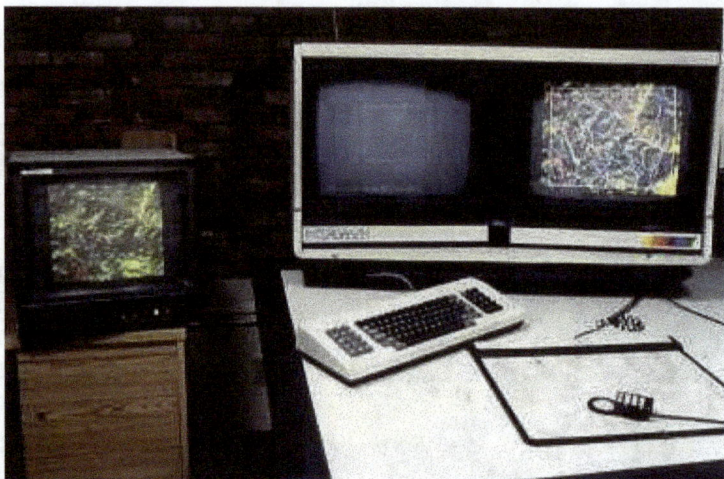

Figure 29: The computer system

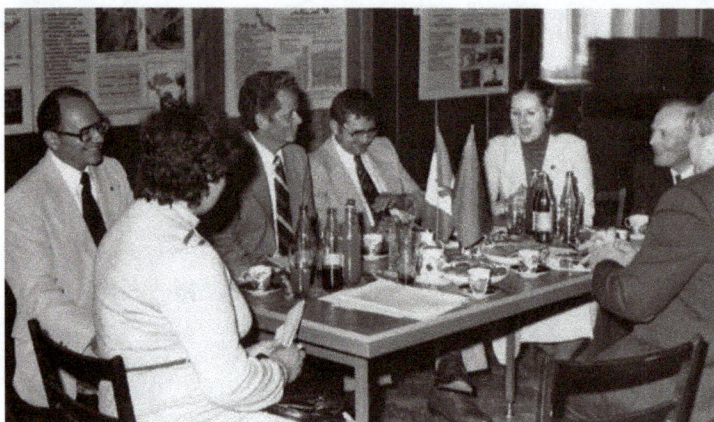

Figure 30: I participated in a delegation to The Soviet Union in 1982

In 1990, I left government work and took a job in the private sector. In my new position, I traveled around the world promoting Canadian business. I opened an office in Hungary, and traveled around Russia, China, and India (I was in India 14 times during the period of 2001-2009). I also had the opportunity to visit many countries, such as The U.S.A., Hungary, Italy, Austria, Romania, The United Kingdom, Switzerland, Malaysia, Kuala Lumpur, Indonesia, Japan, China, and Russia. I was a successful entrepreneur promoting our company, in good health and enjoying life.

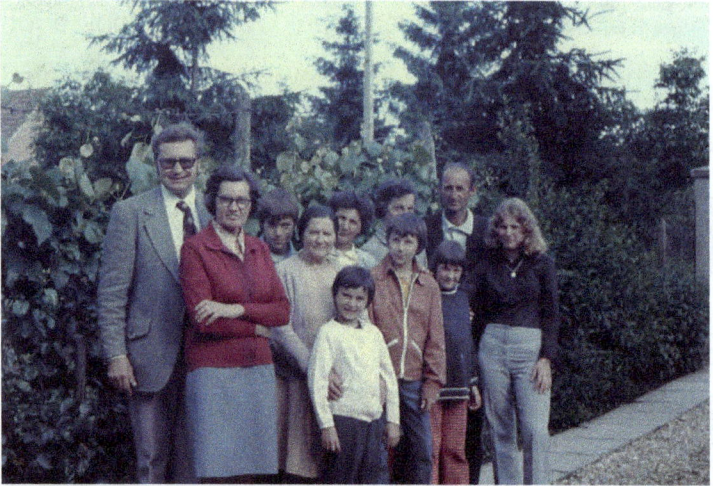

Figure 31. Visiting my relatives in Hungary

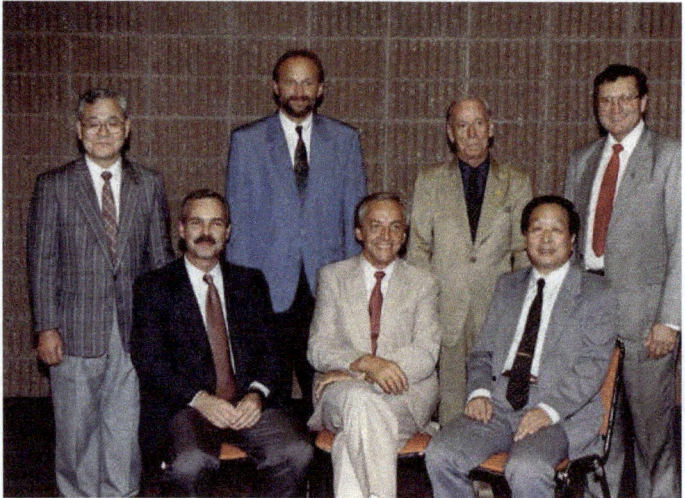

Figure 32. I was elected as Leader of Commission VII

I felt like I was on top of the world. I had enjoyed traveling in my government position; and now I had even greater travel opportunities.

The Executive and Technical Commission Presidents of ISPRS met once a year in different countries. In 1989 we met in Zurich, Switzerland; in 1990 I hosted the meeting in Victoria; the 2001 meeting was held in Glasgow, Scotland; and in 2002 we met in Washington D.C. for the XVII International Congress. Each Technical Commission President was required to organize a mid-term Symposium. I organized the Commission VII Symposium in Victoria, B.C., which was held September 17-21, 1990. Over 240 papers from 23 countries were reviewed by the Scientific Committee and a total of 192 were accepted in four concurrent sessions. There were two plenary sessions, one at the start of the conference on Tuesday morning and the other at its conclusion on Friday. There were also twelve workshops covering the following topics: Geographic

Information Systems (GIS) Concepts; GIS Applications for Management; GIS Applications for Operators; Satellite Image Analysis (SIA) Concepts; SIA Applications for Operators; Photogrammetry and Photo-interpretation Concepts; Aerial Photo Interpretation; Radar Concepts and Applications; Expert Systems and Artificial Intelligence; Remote Sensing for Teachers and Educators; and Environmental Site Assessment and Monitoring. Over 400 international delegates participated in the Symposium.

Each Commission President was charged with organizing Workshops on topics that fell under their specific area of scientific expertise. During my term, I organized 23 different workshops, which were held August 3-14, 1992. Each workshop focused on futuristic technology in the area of Photogrammetry and Remote Sensing; workshop attendance exceeded all expectations. My term as president of ISPRS Commission VII came to an end during the

1992 congress held in Washington, D.C. I was still on top of the world.

PROSTATE CANCER

Then, suddenly, out of nowhere, in January of 2004, I was hit with Prostate Cancer. My family doctor informed me that my PSA reading was high, up to 9.0. She advised me to visit a Urological Surgeon. Then on September 21^{st,} a series of tests later, the specialist told me that I had prostate cancer. This was a real shock for me. I was 66 years old, and I had cancer. When I reached home, I poured myself a strong drink, trying to take in the reality of the situation. I have cancer; I might recover; but, I could die from it. The doctor told me that he could operate, but there was a slight risk that I could end up an invalid. He suggested severing the penis, as the chances are good that I would recover; but, there was a remote chance that I could end up impotent. I thought a lot about the procedure, and declined the operation. The surgeon then sent me to an orthopedic specialist, who described radiation treatment. There were some risks to be sure, but not the same as severing your penis. I opted for this. In January 2005, I started radiation treatment, and completed a total of 35 treatments. One of my neighbours who had also undergone radiation treatment advised me that I would have to be undressed during the procedure. He recommended getting slippers and a dressing gown; this turned out to be a good idea. At least this way I could be comfortable. The radiation was from Monday through Friday at 4:30 pm. This allowed me to work until 3:30 pm before I had to go for radiation treatment. It also gave me the weekends off to recover. During the radiation 35 sessions, I did not miss a single day of work. I did find that radiation schedule exhausting, though and spent a lot of time in bed afterwards, just recovering. I found it all worthwhile because on March 9th, I was informed that my PSA had dropped to 6.5, so I was feeling better. On March 17th I went for a blood test prior to radiation treatment, and it was very painful. When I got home after radiation, I was bleeding heavily and it did not stop for about an hour. That was just a temporary problem, though, and on March 31^{st,} I was given the good news that my PSA count had dropped to 4.64, and on May to 2.72. My most recent PSA level was 0.35, and it has not increased since then.

In 2008 I wanted to have my experiences documented in a book, mainly for my children and grandchildren. So, I wrote a book titled "Dare to Take the Next Step"

Then, in 2009 I published a book with several others called "Death Can Wait" Stories from Cancer Survivors; the other authors were Roslyn Franken, Jacquelin Holzman, and Max Keeping. Each of us is a cancer survivor. Thirty-four cancer survivors were invited to share their experience fighting the dreaded disease. These stories provide insight into the initial reaction people have when they are told, "you have cancer". To some, it felt like a death sentence, while others treated the news as a wakeup call to make changes in their lifestyle.

One of the stories in the book was written by Max Keeping, an anchor for CTV 6 pm news, who had been diagnosed with prostate cancer. The doctors told him that 91 percent of those treated for prostate cancer return to work within about 6 weeks; eight percent return within 4-6 months due to complications. Max considers himself as one of the remaining one percent. His bladder was damaged, which hindered his recovery. He was off for 3 weeks, had a catheter for 9 months, needed 40 hours in a hyperbaric chamber, external radiation, and hormones. After 6 years of treatment, he is finally free of prostate cancer, but he just underwent a 12-hour operation for stomach cancer.

Roslyn Franken, another author from the book, was at a beach party in December 1994. Around 3 a.m., her neck became severely swollen and painful. Biopsy tests revealed a clear case of Hodgkin's Disease, cancer of the lymph nodes. She was in Stage II. Chemotherapy treatment would be administered once every three weeks for the next nine months. The oncologist informed her that side effects of treatment would include hair loss, nausea, fatigue, mouth sores, muscle spasms, back ache, and severe constipation, all of which she experienced to varying degrees. The cancer, however, that seemed at first like an insurmountable setback turned out to be a launching pad to a whole awakening process that caused her to identify and challenge believes, break negative patterns, take risks and try new behaviors. Eighteen years later she is still going strong, author of a new book on The List: 9 Guiding Principles for Healthy Eating and Positive Living; she also is engaged as a professional speaker.

Jacquelin Holzman, another cancer survivor, had just finished 15 years of municipal politics, serving six years as Mayor. Then, in March of 1998, just four months after her term as Mayor ended, she was diagnosed with breast cancer. She fought hard and worked for greater cancer awareness among the general public. She and her daughter have raised over $200,000 dollars for cancer care and research. In addition, hundreds of women becoming more aware of the risk involved, signed up to get mammograms. Greater awareness of the importance of living a healthy lifestyle, combined with increased emphasis on developing new and quicker diagnostics techniques offers hope for the future without cancer.

The 34 other contributors to the book also described their struggle with cancer. Breast cancer (Ductal carcinoma in situ, Invasive Ductal carcinoma, Lobular Invasive, Metastatic Stage, Triple-Negative Inflammatory) was dominant in the group, then Prostate cancer, Hodgkin's disease, Non-Hodgkin's Lymphoma, Esophageal cancer, Colon cancer, Brain cancer, Leukemia, Malignant tumour of unknown origin, Collision tumours, and Colorectal cancer. Since the book was published in 2008, I am sad to report that three of the contributors have passed away. It's a good read because each contributor provides a glimpse into the fears and emotions associated with the disease, as well as how to overcome.

For myself, I saw the doctor in September 2012 and was pleased to be informed that my prostate cancer is resolved, and I do not even have to make a return visit.

MY RECOVERY FROM STROKE

I have been on top of the world, at the top of my game, with a successful academic and professional business career. Then everything changed. First I was hit with prostate cancer and then a stroke. I recovered from prostate cancer relatively smoothly, without missing so much as a day of work. Recovering from a severe stroke is a different story.

In my recovery, I had to study and relearn the simple acts of walking and talking. The first speech therapist, Julia, was very smart and professional. She asked me many questions covering various topics, and I had difficulty finding the words to respond. Even attempting to identify familiar objects in pictures was a struggle for me. I recognized the picture, but could not find the word to describe what I knew I was seeing. Julia would then tell me the word, but I had difficulty remembering it after being told. During the four weeks I worked with Julia, I made very little actual progress. I started out with a 20-word vocabulary, and it was slow progress from there.

The physiotherapist, Chantelle, was most helpful in getting me back to full mobility. She encouraged me to try my best even if it seemed too hard. She put me on the stationary bicycle and had me pedal slowly, and definitely, with the purpose of learning to ride. She understood that I had a problem, that I would slow down and only gradually be able to start back up again. The first time she had me exercise for 20 minutes; then our sessions were increased to an hour. Even though my legs were very stubborn and uncooperative, I did make progress. In fact, Chantelle helped me the most in the early stages of my recovery. I was actually starting to walk again, which made me feel much more confident about getting better.

Well, the toilet training was quit eventful. It took two people just to get me over to the toilet. First, I had to be lifted from the bed to the wheel chair, then on to the toilet with two people assisting me. In the hospital I accepted having to go to bed with undergarments; but felt uncomfortable about it in the rest home. I felt motivated to continue trying even at the beginning, which was an early sign of recovery. Immediately after the stroke, my hands were not cooperating, and people had to do everything for me. At one point, the nursing staff got me to the toilet; and I ended up being left to sit there for over half an hour because I was unable to communicate with staff. It was during that time sitting alone on the toilet that I found the ability somewhere inside me to call them back.

After about a month in the heath unit, the nursing staff and a doctor recognized improvement, and transferred me to The Elisabeth Bruyere Centre. This was extremely good for me: it was a start of the actual rehabilitation process, where I had hoped to recover. The transfer process took about three weeks, which improved my stay in the research centre because I saw the transfer becoming a reality.

During the interim, while waiting for the transfer, I continued improving, especially in physio. Chantelle worked with me, improving my skills. Besides the bicycle, I moved over to the treadmill, where I held myself up using the hand rails and focused on exercising my legs. I began by dragging my legs, one by one, then I slid my legs along while holding myself up with my hands.

On April 29th I asked Rose and the nurses to allow me to leave the hospital premises. With strict instructions not to take me home (stairs), we settled on for the Billings Bridge food court centre. My legs were quite unresponsive still, and Randy and I had to physically lift them into the car. I began to wonder whether a full recovery with full leg mobility would ever be possible. Then Randy left the hospital campus and things looked quite strange to me. I had been inside the hospital for over two months and everything appeared new. Yet, I took hope, thinking of how I was here, actually outside the hospital walls, after the doctor had told my wife I would live the rest of my life as a vegetable. I was thinking what a treat it was just to drive around in the car and go out for afternoon coffee. The drive was soon over, and I had to physically lift my legs out of the car and into the wheelchair. This was more difficult than the reverse, but Randy and I were determined to steer my legs out of the car and into the wheel chair. Even though my right arm was still not working well at all, together we managed to get my legs into the wheelchair. It was a major accomplishment just being in a wheelchair in the food court at Billings Bridge. We went up to the food court, enjoyed a coffee and talked. I felt so proud of my family, and I was out of the hospital. When we got to back to the hospital, I had to get out of the car, into the wheel chair again and then subsequently back into the bed. This was the very beginning of my outings away from the hospital. In May I was able to actually go home every Saturday. My family helped me up the stairs, and the wheel chair did the rest. The first two Saturdays I sat in my wheel chair in my own home, just watching TV and talking to family.

In May I also had to get a haircut. The hospital had a resident barber on the ground floor, and my wife and I made an appointment. We set the appointment for May 19th at 1 pm. The lady barber spent over an hour cutting my hair, which ended up a bit too short, but I enjoyed the experience.

On May 25th we were told that the transfer to Elisabeth Bruyere had been approved, and the ambulance would come in the morning. I was excited about this transfer; I am going to a place where I can focus on recovery. I realize that I still cannot walk; but I will be able to practice with specialists who can help me.

The ambulance picked me up around 10 o'clock and took me to The Elisabeth Bruyere hospital. I was on the fourth floor of the hospital and shared a room with another resident; there was a window so I could look outside.

My physician was Dr. Acharya, who had a good sense of humour and was a very caring person. My RN, Julia, was very patient and attentive in every way. Beverly, the social worker was very articulate and helpful. Terri, the physiotherapist, was the one to actually guide me through my recovery. Isabelle, the occupational therapist, assisted us in getting my home ready for my eventual return. Catherine and Krista, the speech language the rapists had their work cut out for them with my language skills recovery. There was also a dietician named Anita, but I did not see her much. Jasprit, the pharmacist, who I saw often, was always ready with suggestions for me.

The hospital had excellent staff that attended to all of my needs. I knew I was in the process of recovering, slow and gradual, but I was progressing. I noticed others in the hospital complaining about the staff; but mine were excellent; they assisted me with every aspect of my recovery.

Since my first objective was mobility, I was lucky to be assigned Terri as my mobility coach because she provided an excellent program. Because I was unable to stand at the beginning, she provided bicycle training and a specially hand therapy session. As I progressed, she assisted me in learning to walk again, so I could support myself using both my hands and legs. Then, finally, I progressed to exercises that relied only on my legs for support. The results were very encouraging; I could stand on my legs with some support from my hands, and I even tried to walk. My legs were slow to cooperate, but strength did return to my entire leg. I was starting to walk again; I had a long way to go, but it was a beginning.

The occupational therapy room provided objects to manipulate to get coordination right. I did have a problem in this area; my right leg and hand were slow, but responsive. I spent time on the computer using games to get my coordination and my balance corrected.

The speech room, on the other hand, I found very challenging. Catherine was both pleasant and supportive, and with her help I was able to get the words out of my mouth, well most of the time. It surprised me so much to discover how difficult it was for me to articulate the words of familiar pictures I was shown. I did enjoy her classes, but vocabulary returned to me slowly. Krista, on the other hand, was very academic, and I just struggled so much to articulate what I so much wanted to say. Both teachers gave me the impression that learning speech would be a problem for me.

The second weekend I tried to get out for most of the day. This was not a problem as the hospital encouraged me to spend time with the family, and I had a very supportive family. Before leaving I met with the nurse about challenges I might face at home, mainly about do's and don'ts about walking, climbing the stairs, eating home cooked meals and house cleaning tasks. The first home visit was scheduled for afternoon between lunch and supper; it was then increased to lunch, and then lunch and suppers. I had to report back after each visit, telling them which tasks I was able to perform. I found the visits to be quite an undertaking; but, with the help of my family, I was able to strengthen my legs and even do a bit of walking.

Jennifer and her children visited me several times a week, and Ryan and Sara were a lot of fun. Randy visited me every 3 weeks and was very encouraging. Michael came back for a visit on my birthday (June the 9th) and we had a lot of fun. From the 7th to the 12th of June we went out for lunch and supper every day. Well, we over did it because my legs seized up and I couldn't move them at all. Michael helped me up the steps into our house mobility was a bit of problem. He went back to Wisconsin on the 12th and I could not stand the pain I was in. Around 4 pm Rose called the Ambulance, which transported me back to the hospital. The hospital staff was quite concerned, and after being examined by both a nurse and student doctor, I was taken by ambulance to the main hospital. By six p.m., as I was returning to the main hospital, I found that I could not move my legs at all.

Well the hospital gave me a thorough work over. They thought the paralysis had returned and spent two full days examining me from top to bottom. First, they sent me to brain scanning, then kidneys and liver, and finally foot scanning. After two full days, they concluded that my foot was sore and needed to rest. I was, then, sent back to Bruyere to recover.. The nurse was a little upset that I had undergo all of that testing, but it confirmed that I needed medication for my foot. The physio therapist went easy on me for a while and I slowly returned to full scale exercise and walking. By the middle of June, I was doing a bit of walking again.

After this a meeting was held to decide whether I could be released from the hospital or if I would need to stay a while longer. I asked the physio therapist if I could walk with a cane. She encouraged me to try it. I ended up being able to walk around the hospital with the use of a cane, even to my exams. But then I suffered a painful attack of "gout" and had to recover from that. Even having the sheets touch me caused pain. After taking the proper medication, though, I was able to get rid of the gout.

Another meeting was held on June 29th at 11:15 a.m., which was attended by all of my staff, my wife, and me. Unfortunately due to the setback with gout, I was back in the wheel chair again.

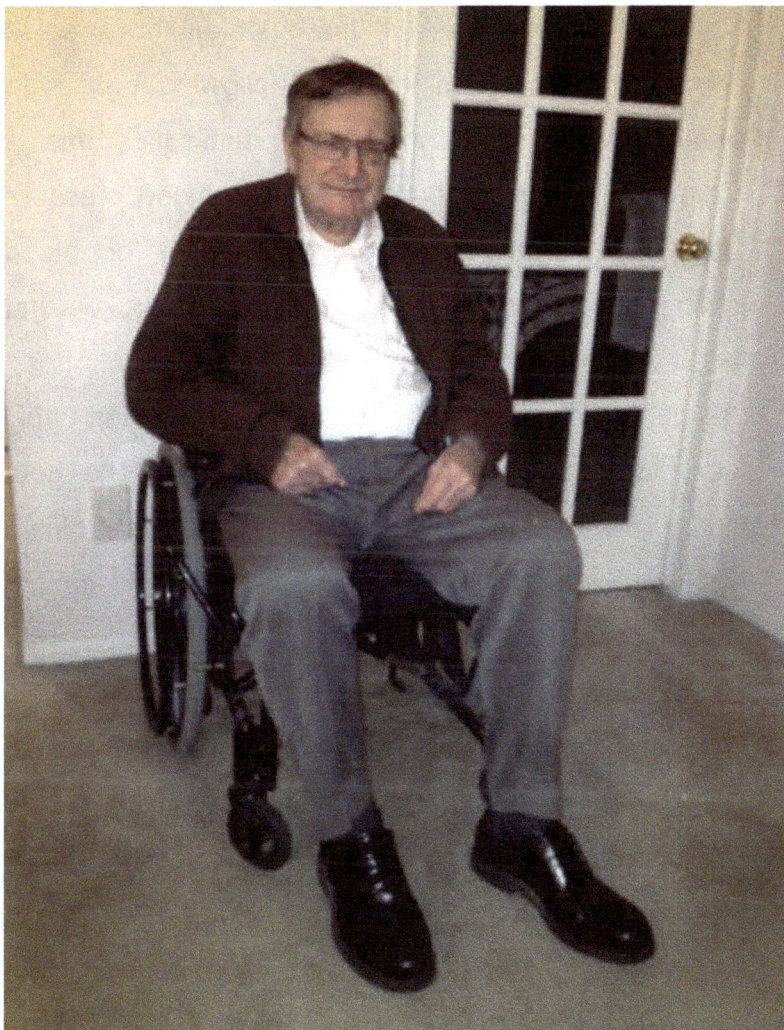

Figure 33. I did not stand up; I wheel chair bound.

Dr. Acharya was the first speaker. She said,: "Mr. Hegyi was admitted here following right side weakness, with communication difficulties arising from a left side cerebral stroke. His blood pressure and diabetes are well controlled. He is on blood thinner medication to protect from future strokes and heart attacks. He had gout flare up which will need regular medication." The doctor's report thoroughly described my present medical condition. The gout flare up was under control, and the diabetes problem was resolved. I was put on blood thinner to control future heart attacks, and my blood pressure was under control. The medication reduced my blood pressure to 105 over 70; previously it was 140 over 95, although at critical times it had risen to 200 over 115. The gout had cleared up too; previously it was all red and swollen and now it was glowing white and healthy. I felt going to live a long life in this new state of good health.

Julia, the nurse, gave the following report: "Mr. Hegyi is pleasant and cooperative. He is on a regular diabetic and cholesterol diet. He can eat independently. He was started on a self-medication program and has advanced to step II." Julia was my favourite nurse, who looked after me regularly and helped me to reach step II in the self-medication program. She assisted me in making my bed, keeping the place tidy, and introduced me to good diet. This was a big help to me in my recovery.

The social worker commented: "Discharge planned for July 6 at 10 am. You have been registered with ParaTranspo and provided information on "helpline personal emergency system" and South East Ottawa Community Support Services". I found the social worker efficient, but super officious. She rarely smiled and made you feel like a member of a brigade. She was, however, super officious and prompt.

The occupational therapist, Beverly, provided the following comment: "Seen 3x1 week to work on right hand function to accomplish bilateral activities. Provided with perceptional/cognitive activities; Montreal Cognitive assessment scored 14/30; difficulty visuospatial/executive function, attention, language, abstraction, and delayed recall. Seen 1x1 week by rehab assistant to work independently with self-care tasks, can dress and wash independently at sink + suspension for shower with appropriate equipment. Home ex. arm/hand program given to patient, list of equipment needed for discharge + vendor list provided". Well I had not understood of lot from the report but everyone was nodding, so I concluded it was OK. A very kind therapist named Beverly helped me to adjust to my at home rehab routine.

The physiotherapist, Teri, wrote: "We have been working on improved movements. Right hand and leg weakened, balance, walking. There is an improvement in all areas. He can walk supported by a cane. I will give you a home executive program with a cane". Of all the therapists, the physiotherapist helped me the most. She taught me to walk and she helped me to become independent again. I will always be grateful to her.

The speech-language pathologist wrote: "We have been working in written expression which has improved. Self-monitoring is better and you are able to correct your own spelling errors more often. With respect to comprehension, this area is strong and only mildly affected. Expression continues to improve; word finding is difficult at times but is improving. I will recommend that he be seen in the outpatient clinic for our present speech pathology services". I agreed with the speech therapist regarding her evaluation, and I was looking forward to continued support in this area. Both speech therapists were helpful and contributed greatly to my overall recovery.

Following the report, we entered the discussion phase. The doctor told me that driving a car is still not possible; and, I would have to take an exam before I could drive again. Following the written test, I would have to take a road test with two instructors: one for the physiological tests and the other one for road test. The occupational therapist come to my home and provide recommendations for improvement in the living environment. The physiotherapist was happy with my progression, and she said that she felt I would be able to walk without a cane in about 6 months. This was good news for me.

The next day (June 30th), the occupational therapist took me home in taxi. I had to prove I could do everything on my own before I could qualify to go home. I was first confronted with the front steps, but was told I could use the railing to support myself while walking up. I passed, and she noted that I was able to use the entrance to my house on my own. I had no problems achieving any tasks related to the living room. I did require assistance with an electronic device in order to get out of my wheel chair, and that was fine. Concerning the kitchen, she said I was able to move around and reach items in drawers, cupboards and the refrigerator. She also noted that I was able to move chairs around the kitchen and dining room, as well as able to transport items from place to place. The bathroom was a challenge: we had to consider purchasing another RTS with arms to facilitate toilet transfers. She did not consider a use of walk in shower at this time as the walk in set up was not ideal. The main bath room had a RTS with an arm, so that was OK. My daughter will provide tub transfers to a bench. We were advised to purchase anti-slip mat for both tubs. The bed room was fine, but she did recommend clearing the floor space near the dresser to avoid risk of a fall. Finally, she did not recommend access for to the basement or back yard. She said that she recommended an effective release date from the hospital of July 6th.

I exercised all week preceding my release date and was packed and ready to be released on July 6th at 10 am. I said my good bye to the hospital staff and thanked them for looking after me. I gave my walking chair back to the hospital, and prepared to exit the hospital using only a cane for support. This was the first time I had done that, and it felt so good. As my wife drove away from the hospital, I was thinking, the "vegetable" is now walking with a cane. I had progressed a lot since the stroke and far surpassed the original doctor's predictions.

It was noon when we got out of the hospital, and I told my wife that I wanted to go to my office after lunch. We had lunch in a Thai restaurant, where I enjoyed my favourite food: mushroom soup, chicken curry, and ice cream. Then, we were off to the office. My office was on the second floor, and I climbed up the stairs with a cane, one step at the time, and made my way to my chair. Of course I was not doing it entirely alone, but I was back in my office. After an hour, I was ready to go home. I told my wife that I wanted to walk into my house un-assisted and sit in my chair. This was one of the most important things for me: It meant that I was truly ready for my home coming. After the car stopped I got out without assistance and walked towards the stairs. I climbed up the 3 steps on my own and headed towards my chair. I sat down unassisted and felt like a million dollars. I had made it home on my own!

And now I was home, walking with a cane, but I was walking. The first evening alone sitting in my chair, I was thinking a lot. After five months in the hospital I was at home and ready for further recovery that lay ahead. I knew there was still a fight ahead of me. I am still partially paralyzed, my speech is only 40 percent of what it once was, and my construction of words still needs improvement. I started my work, however, a little bit each week, and had increased it to full measure my Christmas time.

Following a few weeks at home, I was invited to out-patient activities. Maria, a physio therapist, was the first to invite me. She followed the same protocol as the earlier instructors, but she was more focused on using words to construct a complete conversation. She still used the dictionary to question me, but the lesson was more oriented to everyday conversation. I was actually taught sentences, which I could use in everyday conversation. The main focus course was teaching us how to make conversation. She asked me to make conversation about work or a hobby, and I was assigned the preparation of a sentence on that topic for our next session. As the sessions progressed, I was given more complex tasks, like inviting co-workers to a party or inviting others out on outings. This was important to me as it would help me with my work. By the time Christmas rolled around, I was discharged from the speech therapy sessions.

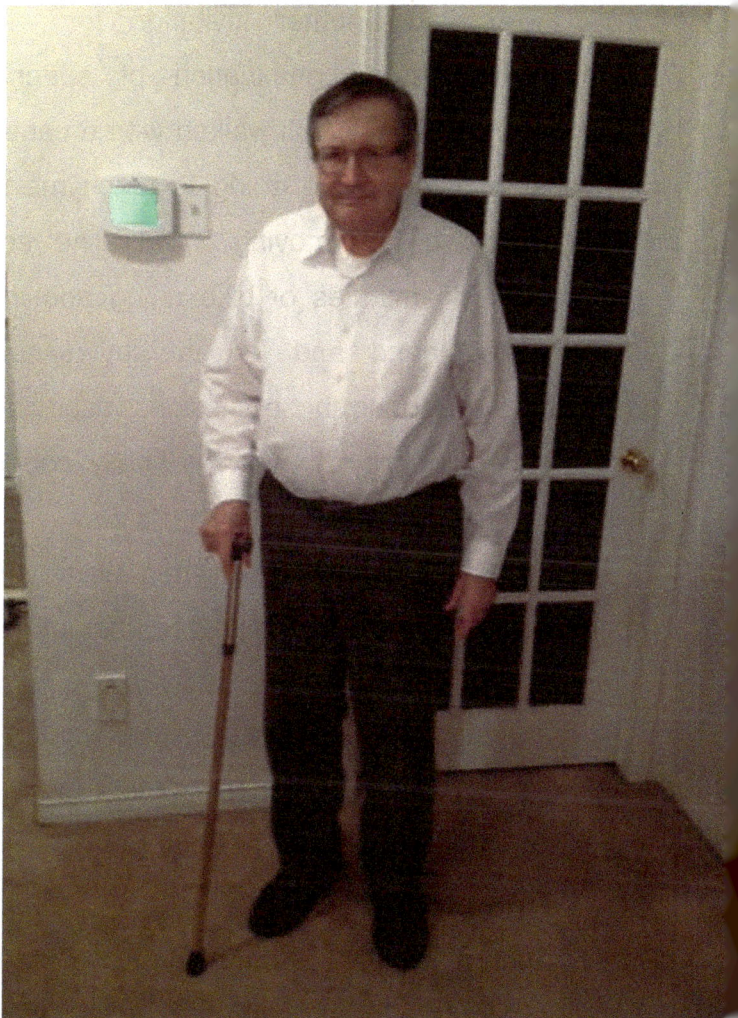

Figure 34. I had graduated to walking with a
cane.

I received another invitation for language therapy. It was a combination of speech and occupational therapy. I still walked with a cane to the sessions, and they were going to teach me how to function in this fast moving world. The sessions started with 15 minutes of bike riding and included individualized hand and leg therapy sessions. I improved a lot during these sessions, especially with arm and leg mobility; they were finally cooperating exactly as they should.

By December I had finished all government sponsored sessions; I had improved a lot, but still had a long way to go before I was entirely back to normal. I started to think about what I would have to do to "get normal" again. By Christmas time I was able to walk without a cane; I was a bit slow, but I was one more step on the road to recovery.

Then my daughter and I had to face a difficult decision together. Right before the stroke I was telling my her that we would take her and the grandchildren to visit their Uncle Mike and Aunt Penny. It was planned as a nice get away for the children because of their Dad passing away; Jennifer was worried about my mobility and my income. I was lucky to get $160 a week in insurance income, and I had enough frequent flyer points for Jennifer, the children and I to travel to Chicago. Jennifer booked the airline tickets, and we left Ottawa on December 22, 2011 bound for Chicago. Jennifer arranged to have Mike pick us up at the Chicago airport, and from there, it was a two hour drive to Madison. The trip went well, I had no motion sickness; an airline hostess helped transport me to the baggage area. Mike was already there waiting, and we got in the car and drove to Madison. About a half hour from the airport we had to stop because Jennifer realized that the children had left a bag behind. So Mike and Jennifer went back to the airport and were able to retrieve the bag while I watched the grandchildren (all alone). When we got to Madison, Aunt Penny and Niece Tasha greeted us with open arms. Just less than a year before I was called a "vegetable"; and now I was walking without even the assistance of a cane. The trip to Madison was very exciting and we did some great stuff. We did lots of window shopping and had nice lunches out; I was also able to take the family to a nice restaurant where you cook your own steaks. Christmas morning was really exciting, opening presents and taking pictures. On Monday morning we drove to Chicago and checked into a hotel. Jennifer and Mike had taken the children to the city and I stayed behind to enjoy a beer and watch TV. Jennifer said the trip to the city was very exciting and they saw a lot of interesting things. The next morning we got up and got get ready for the trip home. We traveled through Montreal to Ottawa, and finally we were home.

Aphasia Centre

In January I started speech therapy at an independent facility called Aphasia Centre. The staff, Gillian, Beth, Helene, Joanne, and Emilia were all professionals in either speech or occupational therapy. At 74 years of age, I was engaged full time in the work of recover, even attending classes for two hours at the Ron Kolbus Lakeside Community Centre in Ottawa on Wednesday afternoons. The attendees are mostly victims of stroke and other related conditions. Their vocabulary is very limited, ranging from about 20 words to about 500. The staff divided the attendees into three or four different groups, placing together individuals of similar language ability.

I continued to work on my English in the speech group, but the progress was slow. Initially, I thought that I would be able to recover all of my pre-stroke language skills, but the progress was so slow. I wanted a swift return to my professional life, which required excellent communication skills, and it just was not happening that way. I had to learn all over again, everything that had once come so natural to me: written language, speech idioms, expressions, mannerisms, and in particular, the culture expressions of the English language. It was very much harder than expected, although it was easier than before I started at the center. I found writing to be even more challenging than spoken language. First, I tried the typewriter, and found it particularly slow and laborious. Even ordinary words were hard to master, and it was much harder than before to remember the spelling. English expressions were very tough to come by, and spelling any words, even everyday ones, was a huge challenge. My language skills had been acquired over time; I had had an entire lifetime to master the language; now, I was trying to re-learn it all at once after an injury to the brain. When I went to work, I got many words confused and found spelling to be just nearly impossible. The scientific parlance that had once come so natural to me was now entirely foreign. Even simple gestures and body language are difficult to master after a stroke. It's like your body just does not know how to perform them anymore. I found this was the most difficult thing for me. Handwriting was even more difficult to master than typewriting; even now I cannot do it with ease. I could re-learn typing on a computer, and after that, it was like my hands and eyes just did not want to cooperate with each other to perform the basic task of handwriting.

When I am to address a group, I find it very difficult to articulate what I want to say. It's as if my brain is just not up to the task of speech generation. You are aware of this, and the delay in your speech can make you nervous. If only the words would come out fluently, then people would more easily understand the point you are trying to make.

From July 6th to the end of the December, I tidied up my office and completed my contract for the Ontario Ministry of Natural Resources. My contract with the Canadian Forces Base was cancelled. In

January 2012, I was trying to get back into research publication. During the five months I was in the hospital research staff in my office were often unable to locate the works they were looking for, which created a situation of no little difficulty. My response to this problem was to clean my office once I was released from the hospital. I brought my books home and erected a new book shelf to house my research materials. I reorganized my research publications and individual studies so that anybody could find it, project by project, and year by year. Then, I attempted to get back into research again at the professional level. I called my contact with the National Research Council and inquired about new contract opportunities. The problem was, I still suffered quite a speech deficit, and I made myself understood only with great difficulty. My mind knew exactly what I wanted to say; but, I was unable to express it properly to the government official.

I guess in the world of research things change slowly, and when it comes to tree growth, it is infinitesimal. So after running a company, I got back into research; in particular I studied the growth and yield of trees. Back In 1970 I had published one of the first articles on tree growth, which focused on the jack pine. Even 40 years after its publication, I noticed my article was still being frequently cited as a reference in other research publications. So I thought a follow up article would be appropriate, covering jack pine tree growth over time. Since I had a good relationship in the staff at the OMNR I asked them to provide me with data covering jack pines and black spruce with 20-year re-measurements. After having the new data, I applied to the Canadian government for funding to analyze the data. My request for funding was approved; and, one year after being released from hospital, I had a contract to complete the research and conduct measurement analyses.

Now, I am in full research work; back in the saddle, publishing again. Over the years I have published around 35 articles, edited a book, and have been invited to speak at major conferences. I have had a career of distinction, and I have been able to sit back and enjoy retirement. I do not, however, want an idle retirement; I want to work at something. So, doing research work and writing books are my retirement projects. I am not ambitious; I had already risen to the top in my profession; now I just want to enjoy my retirement years. At this point in my life, I have had cancer and a major stroke. Recovery meat an entire overhaul of all major body systems. I lost over 50 lbs., and I am in good shape now. I would like to continue my research until I am 80 years old, then I will give it up and focus on writing books.. I look back now at my time in the hospital immediately following my stroke and say, the vegetable is walking and starting a new career.

Losing 50 pounds changed my outlook on life. My appetite has changed; I do not eat the same type of food. Before the stroke, I enjoyed food such as eggs, bacon, sausages, potatoes, T-Bone steak, and all things that tasted good, but were quite fattening. After my release from the hospital I found that my appetite had changed. It is for the better. I still eat eggs, bacon, sausage and T-Bone steaks, but only occasionally. Prior to my hospitalization, I never liked dessert. Now, I love dessert, especially ice cream and pies. However, my body is recovered; I am in perfect health. My blood pressure is normal, the diabetes is under control, and I do not have any other known issues. During my last exam, the doctor told me that I was in perfect health. Every time I get a health report, I cannot help thinking back to the time the doctor in the hospital told my wife that I would be a vegetable.

I am now living healthy, free of pain, and with a much improved outlook on life. I have come to accept that my life will be a continuous process of recovery from the stroke. This recovery process will require a lot of adjusting on my part. First of all, my personality has changed quite a bit. While in hospital, I tried to understand how this had happened to me, how I had ended up a stroke victim. First, I thought it was a sudden attack with no warning and considered my recovery a miracle. But, when I think back now, I realize that I had quite a bit of warning. In December, just before my stroke I had to be hospitalized due to a vein problem in my head. The doctors told me that my heart beat was rising and it had to slow down. This was the first time in my life that I had ever been in an ambulance. I was enjoying the ride; but, when I got to the hospital it was all business. They immediately escorted me to a bed where two doctors examined me. I was connected to many instruments and was given medication to decrease my heart rate. I was in hospital for about 6 hours; and, once my heart rate had recovered, I was released. The following month the same thing happened again. My heart was racing, so I went to the hospital, where they again brought it back to normal. One month later, however, the vein burst in my brain, and so began my struggle against a lifelong vegetative existence.

At this point I am still working to overcome these obstacles and begin a new life. Prior to the stroke I was running a company, but now I had to revisit my options. The company is doing so well, I felt I could focus on research. Yet I still find it difficult to verbally express myself, and writing is tough. I decided to write the book about the Stroke. It was hard at the beginning, just getting on paper what I knew I wanted to say, and finding the right vocabulary was challenging and slow going. As I started to write, I had great difficulty with spelling. For each paragraph, I looked at the dictionary, on average, every five to all the words. Then a few months later, I found I could write almost a page and only consulted a dictionary once or twice per sentence. A few months later, I found I had progressed even further, writing a full page and using the spell checker less frequently. At this point, I can write three to five pages per day, and only require the use of a spell checker every couple of sentences. It has been frustratingly slow, but I found that some of my spelling buddies in the speech group are behind me in spelling, even though they had their strokes two or three years prior to mine. I find writing, though, the toughest challenge to overcome.

Speech therapy, overall, was a major challenge. The words came out slowly, I was stuttering, trying to find the words. During my first sessions of speech therapy at the recreation center, I found that people were at many different stages of recover, some were struggling just to find the word, while others were quite fluent in stringing together entire sentences. We learned a bit more from the sessions when the struggling individuals were mixed in with those who were more advanced. The mixture allowed us to hear proper speech much more clearly.

In August 2012 the Aphasia Centre was relocated to 2081 Merivale Road and some of transferred to the new location. The move was an improvement, and now I was in a group that was much more compatible with my language level. I am now going every Tuesday afternoon.

After the stroke, I re-learned English first, although Hungarian is my native tongue. When I attended a Hungarian party recently with my wife, where mainly Hungarian was spoken, I found it difficult to understand. In a couple of hours, though, the language was already coming back. We stayed over two hours, and my understanding of the Hungarian language was coming back. After the party, I felt even my English speech therapy was improved.

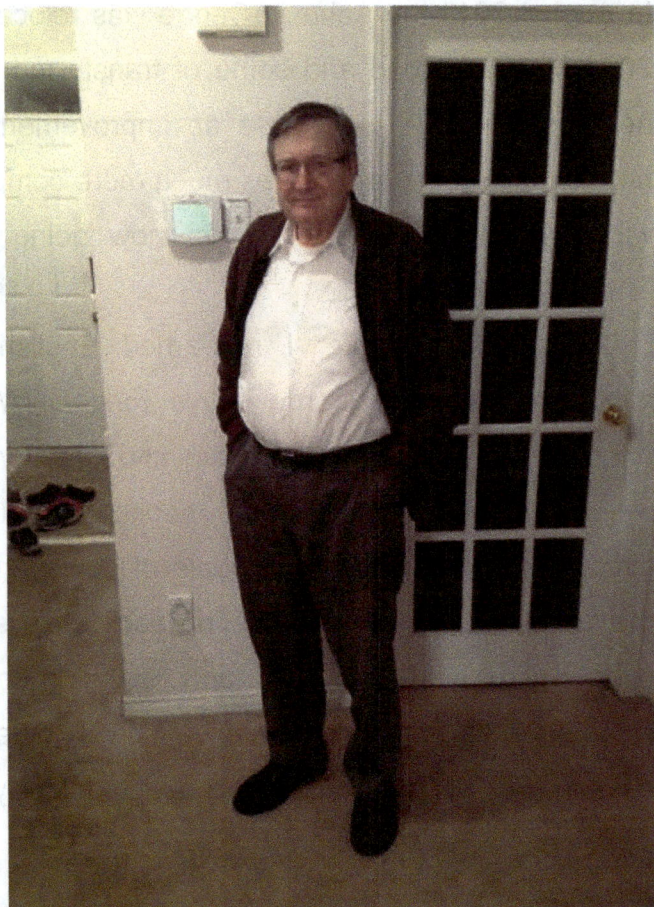

Figure 35. I am waking again, slowly, but I am walking.

RECOVERY WITH SOME ADJUSTMENTS

I am recovering slowly, but I realize now that I will never be the same again. It is January 2013 almost two years after the stoke, and I am still experiencing slow, but steady recovery.

At this point, I have recovered from the paralysis completely (except for two of my fingers, which do not close completely). I do not have a limp or any other physical disability. My hands function perfectly and the paralysis is completely gone.

My speech is about 60 percent cured. I am working to recover the structure of complete articulate sentences. I can definitely say that my speech is returning; and it will be near perfect in about a year or two.

The 50 pound weight loss solved a lot of problems as well. I am relatively thin and feel much better. Of course I take 10 different medications daily, from blood pressure medication and blood thinners to arthritis medication and others. Some movements are still slow, but I am quite strong otherwise. I plan on learning to drive again, but I still need to remove the cataracts from my left eye.

I am now working full time in the office and writing this book about the stroke. I am still speech therapy to further improve my language skills. I have been appointed to the board of the society, and this is a very good thing for my recovery.

My recovery process required adjustments. Even when was unable to communicate at all, I understood the doctor's prognosis. I fought the odds, gaining the ability to walk again, ready to lead a functional life. I started with a 20-wordvocabulary and partial paralysis to about a 1,500 word vocabulary and completely recovered paralysis. Next year I will continue to play golf.

Now, I appeal to my maker to allow me to lead a normal life again. At least for a period of 20 years until my grandchildren have started their careers, and I am truly ready to retire.

Until then, I am going to enjoy my grandchildren. I will watch Ryan play hockey, going every weekend to see him play (I can enjoy it much better now with clear vision after having my right cataracts removed). I will watch my granddaughter playing with her toys, and I will simply enjoy myself.

CONCLUSION

As I recovered from my stroke I found a deep and abiding faith in God. In particular, I had great comfort in the Footsteps in the Sand story.   "God, I believe in you even though I cannot see you. In my dreams as I looked back on my life, I see two sets of footsteps on the beach, most of the times, yours and mine. But, when I was going through difficult times, I only saw one set of footsteps".

And God replied:

"My precious child, when you were going through some difficult times that was the time when I carried you".

www.ingramcontent.com/pod-product-compliance
Lightning Source LLC
Chambersburg PA
CBHW052134270326
41930CB00012B/2881